Robert James Culverwell

Guide to Health and Long Life

Or what to eat, drink, and avoid

Robert James Culverwell

Guide to Health and Long Life
Or what to eat, drink, and avoid

ISBN/EAN: 9783337310226

Printed in Europe, USA, Canada, Australia, Japan

Cover: Foto ©Lupo / pixelio.de

More available books at **www.hansebooks.com**

GUIDE

TO

HEALTH AND LONG LIFE:

OR,

WHAT TO EAT, DRINK, AND AVOID;

WHAT EXERCISE TO TAKE,

HOW TO CONTROL AND REGULATE THE PASSIONS AND APPETITES; AND ON THE GENERAL CONDUCT OF LIFE.

WHEREBY HEALTH MAY BE SECURED, AND A HAPPY AND COMFORTABLE OLD AGE ATTAINED; THAT AT LAST, WHEN OUR CAREER IS CONCLUDED, WE MAY,

"Like ripe fruit, drop
Into our Mother's lap, or be with ease
Gathered, not harshly plucked."—MILTON.

TO WHICH IS ADDED, A POPULAR EXPOSITION OF
LIEBIG'S THEORY ON LIFE, HEALTH AND DISEASE

BY ROBERT JAMES CULVERWELL, M. D.

NEW YORK:
PUBLISHED BY JAMES MILLER,
522 BROADWAY.
1867.

CONTENTS.

CHAPTER I.
On Nervous and Delicate Health 18

CHAPTER II.
How to Live, What to Eat, Drink, and Avoid . . . 26
    Diet 27
    Vegetables 36
    Remarks on Condiments 42
    Liquids 43
    Beer 45
    Wines 46
    Spirituous Liquors 48

CHAPTER III.
Relative Digestibility of Different Articles of Food . 50
    List of Articles of Diet, with the Time required for their Digestion 50
    Cookery 51
    Quantity of Food 52
    Time of Eating 53
Snuffing and Smoking 54
Late Hours 56
Exercise and Fresh Air 58

CHAPTER IV.
On the Passions 64

CHAPTER V.
Summary 70
    Diet and Regimen, with Remarks 78

CHAPTER VI.
Dietetic Rules 83
    Low and Middle Diet 83
    Special Diet, for a Nervously-Debilitated Invalid . . 85
    Full Diet 86
    Milk, Farinaceous, Vegetable, and Fruit Diet, and Directions for making Curry 87

CHAPTER VII.
Liebig's Theory on Life, Health, and Disease . . . 89
    Summary of the Liebigian Theory 97

CHAPTER VIII.
Remarks on Bathing Generally 103
    Warm Bathing 103
    Vapor, Sulphur, Fumigating, and other Bathing . . 107
    Cold Bathing 108

PREFACE

TO

THE AMERICAN EDITION.

We have much pleasure in presenting a re-print of a work, of which some 60,000 copies are sold annually in England ; and at a price which will bring it within the reach of every individual within the United States. It is probably the best work on Health and Long Life ever published.

It is well said, by one who had thoroughly studied the subject, that the highest ambition of an ancient Greek was to be healthy, beautiful and rich. We cannot help thinking that the old Athenians, in this respect, were wiser than ourselves. Much as we boast of our wonderful intelligence, we have not yet practically attained to a method of life so comprehensive as that pursued, not only by philosophers, but by the men of fashion about town in Africa and the Peloponnesus. They placed health first, and money-making last, while we invert this order. Yet they were Pagans, and we Christians. Surely we should cry "shame" to ourselves.

In reality, the two principal objects sought by the ancient Greek, health and beauty, were but one and the same. For beauty cannot exist without health. The man who is constantly confined at the counting desk soon acquires an habitual stoop ; the one who devotes his whole soul to money-making becomes wrinkled before his time. On the contrary, he who indulges in proper exercise and recreation, as, for example, a well-to-do farmer in healthy districts, carries an erect frame to the verge of seventy, and has a ruddy cheek even when an octogenarian. The first, by neglecting the laws of nature, not only destroys his own manly bearing, *but transmits a puny form and weakly constitution to his children. The last perpetuates a race of hardy sons and majestic daughters.*

There is but one way to preserve the health, and that is to live moderately, take proper exercise, and be in the fresh air as much as possible. The man who is always shut up in a close room, whether the apartment be a minister's study, a lawyer's office, a professor's laboratory, or merchant's gas light store, is defying nature, and must sooner or later pay the penalty. If his avocation renders such confinement necessary during a portion of the year, he can avoid a premature breaking down of the constitution only by taking due exercise during the long vacations of the summer and winter months. The waste of stamina must be restored by frequent and full draughts of mountain and sea-beach air, by the pursuits of the sportsman, by travel, or other similar means. Every man who has felt the recuperative effects of a month or two of relaxation, knows from his own experience how genial its influence is; how it sends him back to business with a new flow of spirits; how it almost recreates him, so to speak. Between the lad brought up to physical exercises in the invigorating open air, and one kept continually at school, or in the factory, there is an abyss of difference, which becomes more perceptible every year, as manhood approaches, the one expanding into stalwart, full-chested health, while the other is never more than a half-completed man.

The advantages of exercise are as great in females also. All that we have said about preserving health in the man is as true of the opposite sex. But this is not the whole. The true foundation of beauty in woman is exercise in fresh air. No cosmetics are equal to these. The famous Diana of Poictiers, who maintained her loveliness until she was near sixty, owed this extraordinary result, in her own opinion, to her daily bath, early rising, and her exercise in the saddle. English ladies of rank are celebrated, the world over, for their splendid persons and brilliant complexions, and they are proverbial for their attention to walking and riding, and the hours spent daily out of doors. The sallow cheeks, stooping figures, susceptibility to cold, and almost constant ill-health, which prevail among the American wives and daughters generally, are to be attributed almost entirely to their excessive sedentary life, and to the infirmity caused by the same life on the part of their parent. A woman can no more become beautiful, in the true sense of the term, or remain so, without healthful exercise in the open air, than a plant can thrive without light. If we put the latter into a cellar, it either dies outright or refuses to bloom. Shall we wilt our sisters, wives or daughters by a similar deprivation of what is as necessary to their harmonious development?

In another aspect, the care of health is a more important thing than is usually supposed. There is no doubt that, as between city and country, the population of the former suffers most from want of exercise and fresh air, and that consequently the stamina, so to speak, of a city population is inferior to that of a rural one. It is even said that in some cities, Paris for instance, few strictly town-bred families last over a century, and that, if the population was not continually recruited from the country, it would die out. It is an equally striking fact, and one that lies within the observation of all of us, that the most energetic merchants generally, in New-York, Boston, and Philadelphia, have been originally lads from the rural towns or counties, whose well-balanced health has not only produced well-balanced, vigorous, enterprising minds, but enabled them to endure an amount of fatigue which the average of their city-bred competitors could not rival.

The public weal, therefore, as well as the happiness of the individual, is concerned in this question of health. Yet we Americans almost ignore it, and practically neglect it entirely. The old Greeks had their gymnasiums for physical exercise, which were as much state institutions as common schools are now. Were not the Greeks wiser, after all, than we are, at least in this particular?

INTRODUCTION.

> "How best the fickle fabric to support
> Of mortal man; in healthful body how
> A healthful mind the longest to maintain."

Such is the text and such the purport of the following pages; not to enter into a long exposition of the principles of life, or to describe the very many diseases of the human body, nor to present a collection of remedies for the cure of every trifling twinge, but to submit, in a popular and intelligible form, what seems to be either very little attended to, or very little understood, by the great mass in this commercial and increasing country;—a review of the more probable causes and provocatives, together with the character of many of the ordinary and uncomfortable feelings of ill-health, that harass our existence; conditions somewhat difficult to apply a name to, but which more or less almost universally prevail, and which although not positively and immediately destructive to life, are certainly powerfully inimical to its enjoyments; and also, in a like common sense manner, to point out how much the restoration to health, and the maintenance and prolongation of life itself, depend upon the observance of the simple laws of nature—laws which permit an extensive latitude for personal comfort and indulgences, and are merely opposed to the extravagances and excesses of acquired and vitiated wants—laws relating less to drugging and physicking the body, than to the simple observances of *how to live, what to eat and drink, and when to leave off; how to act, how to think*—in fact, *how to regulate the whole conduct of man, as relates to his health from boyhood to old age*, is the object of this work.

In this category I purpose confining my considerations to those disturbances which find their way through the abuse of the stomach and the senses.

I have lived long enough to arrive at the conviction, that every man has his own life in his own keeping, apart from the contingencies of mortality; that is to say, it rests with himself, by controlling and regulating his appetites, moral and physical, whether he shall secure absence from bodily uneasiness, and attain the full period of his days, or whether, on the contrary, he shall be always ailing, always ill, and unfit to go about his business, a burthen to himself, a trouble to his friends; and, lastly, whether he shall be clipped off in the prime of his existence.

I am, of course, presuming that he be originally perfect in his organization, and, like a good ship, requires but a good steersman to guide him through the perils of his voyage. Unhappily many of our troubles are born with us—indeed there are few new-comers into this world without a blemish; but, thanks to the reparative power within us, sickly constitutions can be improved, hereditary ills diverted, and life protracted and healthily preserved. Who has not heard of Lewis Cornaro, who scarcely, till he was forty years of age, knew what freedom from sickness was, and yet after that period, by strict observance of the laws of animal economy, reached in comfort and happiness the patriarchal age of nearly one hundred years.

Every day presents similar instances in private life of individuals who have by dint of free living, dissipated habits, and great wear and tear, brought themselves to "death's door," but who also, by timely reformation, have recovered tone, and are living instances of healthy and delightful old age. In the onset of our career we commit many errors, seemingly of no importance, beyond the inconvenience of the flitting moment, but which after-experience and reflection tell us may be likened to so many "nails driven into our coffin."

It is said—

"Who never fasts, no banquet e'er enjoys;
Who never toils or watches never sleeps;

and it might be added—

> Who never ails, health never knows.

And verily it would appear that health can only be properly estimated when sickness comes upon us, or when we have bitterly felt its inconveniences; else such outrageous neglect of ordinary precautions, and such acts of wanton excesses, as we see continually being committed on the right and the left, could never be practised; for, sooner or later, the consequences inevitably follow; and then man begins to repine at suffering what he is ready to declare he could not foresee and did not anticipate. It may seem very gratuitous for a medical man to uphold the advantages of temperance and forbearance, as contributive to the preservation of health, and to denounce feasting and drinking, and turning night into day, as sure leaders of evil, by which very evil he finds his occupation and his profit; but the advice may be good notwithstanding; the repueation of the surgeon is not built upon how many legs he may am putate, but upon the many he may save, and reputation sometimes is profit. The public, I dare say, will not complain;—

> "To know thyself's the best insurance thou canst have
> 'Gainst ills that easier prevented are than cured."

But as time may be wasted in reading as well as in writing, and as moralizing, except it be practical, counts to little good, I will at once proceed to carry out the idea started in the onset, *i. e.*, to consider what to avoid and to shun—how best to escape from the dangers to be enumerated—how also to support, to nourish, to exercise, and to preserve in good tone, the fickle frame of man—how to secure the *mens sana in corpore sano*, whereby to live shall be a delight—to breathe a pleasure—to think a luxury—to sleep be rest—and to do good, be our end and aim.   R. J. C.

GUIDE
TO
HEALTH AND LONG LIFE.

CHAPTER I.

ON NERVOUS AND DELICATE HEALTH.

This is a comprehensive phrase, as it embraces all those conditions where a man is "ill at ease." I do not mean to assert that it constitutes every illness under the sun, but it may be relied on as forming the majority of infirmities which hazard not the immediate destruction of life, but which embitter it sometimes beyond endurance. Disease assails us in a variety of ways, but there is not one form which does not more or less involve the disturbance of the general health. The great perils of humanity are indigestion and nervousness. By the former is meant that state of the stomach where the food is not properly, kindly, and satisfactorily disposed of; and by the latter is meant that state of mind and bodily feeling where the being, as before remarked, is "ill at ease." Much as we are in the habit of complaining of this state of things, it is well it is as it is, else we should commit greater excesses than we do. Were it not for indigestion, where would be the limit to our appetites?—and were it not for nervousness, where would be the limit to our indulgences and sensualities? It is transgressing beyond the line which nature has drawn between right and wrong, as a little reflection can demonstrate, that incurs the penalty of bodily and mental suffering. By nervous and delicate health, therefore, I mean that state of mind and body which is comprehended in *mental and physical enervation, in the absence of those attributes and sensibilities, and that vigor of frame and nerve, which characterize the healthy aud well-organized individual; which are also evidenced by the accumulation of those morbid, nervous, and dyspeptic symptoms that harass and distress the possessor, unfit him for the common duties of social aud domestic life, and, ivy-like, cling to the stem they surround.*

This enumeration includes a vast amount of grievances, to the endurance of which death were almost preferable ; but surely it will be consolatory to know that the accumulation may be swept away, ay, at one fell swoop, merely by an avoidance of the causes which produce them—at least, the promise thus held out is worth the experiment.

I am personally acquainted with a gentleman who, up to forty-one years of age (and I have known him for nearly twenty years), never enjoyed good health. He was a dyspeptic, with every bad symptom—continually tormented with flatulence, uneasiness of the head, excessively irritable, and subject to great irregularity of the bowels ; he was a bad sleeper, nervous to a degree, and desponding beyond measure. By merely adapting his diet to his capacity, and altering his habits to something like rationality and consistency, he recovered in less than a month, and now enjoys the most perfect health.

How many younger instances could I adduce, where care and attention supplanted indifference and neglect and where the result was an immediate riddance of growing ailments that were fast overwhelming their victims ; the change was as easy as getting rid of an old garment. *We are not born to die before our time —we are born to live our time out :* we all start (those who are well born) with the elements of old age within us, and there is no reason why we should not attain it, if we only take ordinary care of ourselves.

Such, however, is the sympathy in the human frame, that not the slightest evil can occur without compromising the function of the digestive organs, more or less, and also that of the brain ; and without particularizing any specific symptom wherein careful living may prove of service, I will comprehend all, and insist that there is no one form of complaint, of whatsoever kind, and however contracted, in which careful and prudent living shall not be found, if observed, of a salutary and health-restoring tendency. But before I proceed to that part of my subject, I will offer a prelude in the form of an analysis of the most prominent *causes* of ill health— causes of man's own producing—of the causes of that condition which predisposes the human frame to the most ordinary attacks of disease that are to be seen enumerated in the hebdomadal bills of mortality, and of the causes which directly derange the animal economy, thwart its purposes, and prevent man becoming the dignified being after his Maker's image.

I have said that many of our ills are born with us, that we are ushered into the world with "sorrow in our laps," thanks to those who own us as offspring. These things have been, and it is to be feared ever will be. To those, then, thus already sickly constituted, or those who may so become, I especially address myself: it is hard that to live shall be a struggle; and harder that the terms of so existing shall be so infelicitous to follow, wherein every sense is to be contracted, and every wayward wish to be denied. There is, however, no alternative. There is less pity due to those endowed with frames well toned, and who seem to war with their nature, and by precocious and ill-timed extravagances, triumph—if such their acquirement of a broken-down constitution may be considered—over their better part.

Fortunate, indeed, is he who has nothing to repent for; but where is he to be found? Who does not recollect how much folly he has been guilty of at one time or another of his life? Let him go back to any of the feasts and gorgings he has been present at, and let him bring to his recollection what he consumed on the occasion, and will he not wonder how his stomach could have borne it? The mixture of solids and fluids, and the quantity of both, and the many repetitions? The ghost of these doings would make a formidable regiment. Let him not forget, also, the time he has devoted to the said amusements; the encroachments upon his nights; let him contrast his present feelings with the past; and if he be one who has had his share, will he not exclaim, "Humph! I could not do the same now!" Can any other interpretation be put upon such a confession than that he is now suffering from the effect of them? A twelvemonth of town dissipation in a young man seemingly adds ten years to his life. My own experience as an observer (and who has not now and then been a *particeps criminis?*) reminds me of the extraordinary indulgences, if such they can be called, that have been persisted in by young men, just off on their journey in life. A youth at twenty will dare what a man at forty would dread;—the steaming and savory suppers; the dishes of lobster salads, and oysters in their season; the steaks and chops; the tripe and onions; even to the "baked potato"—the very thoughts and recollections conjure up feelings of envy toward the apparently happy, eager, and juvenile consumers; but the morrow is a sad tell-tale! It might be less were the appetite content with the supper; but the grog and the cigar, and

Heaven knows what else, which follow, are essentials, without which the evening would not be satisfactorily concluded. Even a winter spent in dissipation of this kind plays the deuce with a young constitution. The living alone, the smoking and drinking, and the late hours, apart from the licentiousness—which is a species of extras with young hands generally—often lay the foundation of a permanent dyspepsia. What shall be said, however, of the latter practice—these extras? I address this little publication to men of the world, and especially to the younger; I do not profess it to be suitable for the drawing-room table—I would prefer it should be selected as the closet companion of the reader in search of truth—"the whole truth, and nothing but the truth;" and therefore, what they do not blush to commit, it is not likely they will feel abashed at being told the consequences of. It is a maxim with myself and many others, especially medical men, that it is absurd to condemn all those frivolities, pastimes, and indulgences, simply because we can not partake of them ourselves, and to preach up morality and denials to young blood; but it is equally ungenerous to withhold what our own experience has taught us is the sure result of these said pursuits being carried out to excess; and it may be relied upon, that a great portion of the bodily miseries of human life have their origin in the dissipation and licentiousness of early days. The reader will not suppose that bad habits are only picked up at theatres and taverns; every house has its private sin—every cupboard its poison. The home parties, the friendly visitings, the public feasts, even to the lonely corner in a city dining-room, can engender as much mischief by an abuse of the goodly things presented, as where the senses are led on by gay associations and bacchanalian saloons.

I might go on relating an infinity of comparisons, and give innumerable illustrations in support of my assertion; but we need only look around, and we shall scarcely fail to find, among our companions or in the junior branches of the families we may be acquainted with, one or more individuals, broken up in health from the aforenamed causes. We are all apt to talk of the uncertainty of life; it is true, it is uncertain, but only rendered so by our very transgressions. Scarcely a breafast passes by, but we read of the sudden demise of an old friend or associate; but if we happen to have been acquainted with his habits or his history, we can pretty nearly account why he was prematurely taken from us. At all events we must rest assured there was a cause for it, although we may not be able accurately to detect it. It is remarkable that, notwithstanding we quake and perhaps shudder at the loss, and innately resolve, at the moment, to live immensely careful, the next day undoes our resolves, and we in our turn, sooner or later, afford occasion for the same reflections to our survivors. But more of this in its proper place.

The first irruption to health is usually a disturbance of the stomach. Indigestion may commence in the earliest periods of infancy ; there, however, the fault rests not with the patient but the nurse, and probably the onus may remain at the doors of those who ought to regulate our supplies, until we are sent forth to seek our own fortunes. Early gormandizing, stuffing of sweets, and late hours, tend much to weaken the digestive organs of life. A greedy child seldom makes a healthy man. Children, in fact, should have a diet suited to their juvenile stomachs—should have an appropriate table to themselves, and should keep appropriate hours ; whereas, where the circumstances of the family forbid a separate table, and command not many attendants, the same fare and the same hours serve for young and old. Mixed dishes, rich soups, confectionary, strong drinks, staying up late at night, neglect of exercise, and a residence in a close and confined atmosphere, engender the germs of future discomfort and disease, as surely as the grain deposited in the field yields, in due course, its natural produce. These pecadilloes may succumb, however, to a few surfeits ; and an illness or two causes the mother to be more careful, till the stripling is packed off to school, or arrives at what are called years of discretion, when, possibly, he is left to shift for himself. A fire or a flood has a beginning—so has a complaint. Death rarely visits us without some premonitory symptoms, any more than the flames burst forth, or the waters rise, without a previous, albeit short warning ; and there are few forms of failing health but may be traced to incautious or reprehensible conduct. Hence the majority of the class of maladies I am considering take their origin in early life. Hard and coarse, or rich and sumptuous living, excessive fatigue, in-door imprisonment, or loose abandonment and unchecked idleness ; small tipplings and stolen smokings, or downright drunkenness and an everlasting tobacco breath, all tend to bring about the state of health in question. These phenomena constitute a powerful array of provocations ; but there is yet another underplot of as vast a magnitude, and of as deadly a tendency, which to omit mention of were neglecting the most important duty in the task I have assigned myself. In the preceding remarks, it will be perceived that I have alluded chiefly to those complaints which find their way through the stomach. Man is not merely an eating animal, and consequently there are other ways of wasting life than by overworking the stomach. It were a curious inquiry to seek to know how the abuse of the separate powers of the body can derange the whole, or bring our days to a premature termination; but *it does*, and we must be content to go along with the progress of the times, and catch our information as it comes. However, when we consider the numerous mental and corporeal operations which all play their part, the overtaxing of any single one influencing the whole community of its kind, the reference to a pernicious and demoralizing infirmity presently to be made, will strike the least reflecting observer with its importance. In another part of this work, I offer a brief survey of the proper ties, offices, and influences of the passions. Anger, the extremes of grief and joy, domestic and worldly anxieties, severally excite and injure; nor are the various emotions of a tender character without their salutary or withering consequences. The too early development of any of these feelings, particularly the latter, in its worst sense, constitutes a source of disease little dreamed of. It would be fastidiously ridiculous to suppose that the advanced juvenile, much less the adult portion of mankind, are so ignorant of the grand purposes of life, whereby the great globe is peopled, and civilization kept together, though it is not yet awhile recognized as a fit subject for discussion by the elderly and sedate; and although reference to a topic on which I purpose placing great stress, and am anxious to draw particular attention to, may cause a fluttering among many of my sensitive readers, the perusal of a few pages onward will convince them, that, notwithstanding it shall require delicate handling, its importance must not be overlooked; and therefore, if the flush of modest indignation spring up, the author must be willing to bear the castigation, but at the same time he would supplicate a few moments' attention.

There are other kinds of depressing habits, besides free living and intemperance—besides rioting and the common vices of street and tavern life—besides the devotion to hard study or hard work, or the addiction to perpetual pleasure-seeking—besides the unreined indulgences commenced by the votaries of licentiousness and dissipation, scarcely with the down of manhood on their chin—I mean the still earliest delinquencies of the youthful sensualist, acquired possibly before his palate may have known else than the taste of water, or his thoughts have strayed from the belief that the other sex differed from himself, but who, on the initiation or discovery of the new-found pleasure, knows no limit to its gratification This delusive infatuation is *personal sensuality*. Reader, if you have skipped my preface—if you have miscalculated the purport of these pages—if you be past the age when the consideration of it can concern you, or if a new light break in upon you and you learn, for the first time, that you have wandered from the right road to health—do not commit these leaves to the flames—do not follow the fashion of condemning what may have intruded itself irreconcilably to your feelings, nor feel aggrieved at the monitor that meets your eye ; and if happily it have nothing to reprove you for, content not yourself that the rest of the world is as blameless as you may be. Your own experience, I should say—I mean your observation of others—must convince you to the contrary. The evil does exist, and most fearfully does it prevail ; if, however, it were unattended with any injury to health, all this tirade might be unnecessary, might indeed be considered obtrusive, might be looked upon as impertinent ; for surely what is practised in quiet—what is unseen—can offend no one, else many of the other habits of life might shock the delicate and refined ; but alas! the injury is not only of the passing hour, it is of the age to come, and it is fitting that if the deluded be careless of themselves, they have no right to inflict injury on their successors.

Many will argue and say—" Oh, it is of no moment—besides, boys will be boys, and all the vigilance in the world will not prevent 'this sort of thing,' and why should we trouble our heads about other people's business ? Let them find out the evil of it—our fathers did not forbid us, and the world has lasted a long time and may go on, without our making all this bother about those who are to follow us. Talking of making people chaster, why there never was a time in which so much licentiousness prevailed as at the present moment, and despite all you can do, you cannot alter nature." Now, there are many persons who talk and think in this way ; and although they may here and there be right as to the result, that all our efforts to reform or correct many youths may be next to fruitless, it does not follow that we should not endeavor to do it. Within my knowledge, I can tell of individuals of all ages giving way to this habit, by and from ignorance of its mischievous effects.

The evil I am speaking of has its commencement in earliest life. The secret is acquired by example, or not unfrequently is disclosed by a *liaison* of nature herself. Sooner or later, however, if untaught, it forms part of the natural impulses, and is developed with growing years. The act, which is afterwards resorted to, holds such fascinating influence over a youthful mind, that the culprit conceives he has discovered the climax of earthly enjoyment, and hermitizes himself on every occasion for its realization. The maturer mind, yet unacquainted with its desolating tendency, and whom fear, prudence, or ineligibility, forbids sharing his fortunes and his happiness with a suitable companion, hails it as the refuge for the destitute; and gradually prostrates his dignity in the homage of his baseness. They say the best way of reproving vice is to condemn it in ambiguous terms; for to speak out only instructs the not yet influenced. As good wine needs no bush, truth needs no apology. Better even let the author and his pages, wherein are portrayed the crime and consequences, be discarded and condemned by the over-pure, than that one youthful mind be denied beholding in the mirror here presented the folly of his ways. The ill-nature of the hypercritic will fall harmless, whereas the benefit accruing to the wanderer will save a life of bitterness and sorrow.

The sinfulness of falsehood, of idolatry, and of crime, was tableted on stone, and exhibited on the mount to the righteous and the renegade; and shall a violation of the compact which ties man to his posterity, between nature and her children, of not less enormity, escape rebuke or not be forbidden? It is the stumbling-block of nine-tenths of man, and (why should the charge be withheld;) not a few of woman-kind; it is the secret worm that gnaws at the heart—that saps the trunk of its sustenance, and robs the soul of its nobleness and godlike power; and shall we, generation after generation, hide our knowledge of this demon poison, blush to admit our cognizance of its existence, and suffer it to go on undermining the sapling mind of man, and blast the else luxuriant produce before the meridian of existence be arrived at?

It is an ill province to censure, a better and more pleasing one to console, but a far more useful one to forewarn and advise. A young but humble patient of mine, who was suffering from the unbridled excesses of youth, on seeking my assistance, thus wrote to me:—" My parents had me taught the church catechism—it was their aim to make me an honest lad, and encourage me in my duty to my superiors, but they omitted to instruct me in my duty to myself. My father was an intelligent but poor man, had undergone in his early days all the excitements of a London life, and could not be ignorant of the besetting temptations of youth; but, strange to say, never, as I grew up, gave me five minutes' advice on the subject which has brought me to this state of debility and wretchedness." This case is not a singular one; for although a father may not countenance vicious habits in his son—may not set an example of intemperance and waywardness at home—it is too much to calculate that a young man can escape the contaminations of bad associates, unless continually forewarned of the consequences. Be frugal, steady, and temperate, is the admonition of most parents; but it is the closet chit-chat, the unreserved explanation of wherein really consist the dangers that surround young people which is most needed, and is the most rarely given. Nor is this folly confined to the simple, ignorant, and humble lad. Even the high born, the classically-educated youth, the collegian, the offspring of rank and fortune, is as much, I would say more, addicted to the habit than his less fortunate brother. In my particular branch of practice, my experience has convinced me that there is no exemption from the general charge, and I verily believe that not one individual in a hundred can conscientiously assert his entire innocence of it.

It is not my intention here to enter into a detail of the phenomena which speedily show themselves, and betray the young sensualist—that I have done elsewhere, and to which I shall presently more particularly refer. The object of these passing sketches has been principally to point to the evils—to provoke a reflection upon them—to present them hand in hand with the subsequent suggestions, perhaps considered by some more appropriately termed "Guide to Health and Long Life"—to show, not only how to procure health, but how to avoid getting ill. It is oftentimes much easier to prevent a fire than to put one out, did we but foresee the danger.

In my definition of ill health, I have described it as characterized by general mental and bodily prostration, and as attended with all those symptoms which accompany a disordered or weak stomach, or which is perhaps better understood by the term indigestion; but there are an infinity of symptoms denominated NERVOUS, which occasion nine-tenths of the distress of those who may be designated to be in delicate health : these are the symptoms that more especially mark the career of the victim of sensuality, and which harass his life to a burthensome degree.

Writers of those obscene publications christened by catching titles, with appended announcements of their authors possessing the philosopher's secret of grinding old young again, and restoring pristine vigor to man in his second infancy, attribute every mortal infirmity to the one error in question. They threaten consumption, atrophy, raving madness, and all the horrors of worldly suffering to the deluded who DO NOT consult them, and they promise regenerated life, herculean strength, and unalloyed felicity, to those who DO, and they guaranty (!) to secure the transition from death's door to their promised paradise in as brief time as one week enters another.

Although they draw a most harrowing picture, and their motive is evident, to intimidate the newly-affrighted patient into a compliance with their extortionate demands, still the consequences they describe arising from the practice have at least some foundation in truth. That licentiousness is bodily destructive, as well as mentally annihilative, when carried to the excess it is known to be, there is no doubt. In describing nervous and delicate health—in defining it as marked by mental and physical enervation—by stunted growth and impeded development of the better faculties of man, and by the presence of those feelings which strip life of its charms, and all, more or less, arising from careless and dissipated living, and personal indifference or total disregard of the common expectancies or dues of life, the picture were faintly drawn were such to be described as the ONLY consequences of THE one fault. If the divinity of thought, the nobleness of bearing, and the supremacy of manhood, depended upon organization, not the least cause of structural deficiency may be attributed to the sensualist of the past and present race of man. What secrets could the sequestered chamber, or even the devotional cloister unfold, had walls but tongues!

Such are a few of the prevailing errors of early and single life. Ill health pays us a visit at all ages, but the epoch of puberty is the most dangerous. It is at this period generally that a young man is initiated into a new life; he rejoices in slipping the noose of his mother's apron-strings, and doing for the first time all that becomes a man. It is at this period he acquires the relish for convivial society, enters the oyster-cellar, and speedily falls a proselyte to its enticements. The vice of the delusionists is engrafted generally earlier, and is continued with unremitting zeal until his new companions or his newly-begotten confidence introduces him to the other sex.

Here new excitements, new pleasures, and new disasters, await him; we will even take it for granted, that his health hitherto is not much despoiled, that he plays the gallant successfully, and is delighted at his new manifestation of manhood. These are but errors common to all of us—still there is scarcely a young man to be found, who ventures forth in search of indiscriminate gratification, who is not sooner or later entrapped in the meshes of his imprudence, and involved, more or less deeply, in the consequent disease common to promiscuous association.

We will pass over to the next feature in our history, to that of married life. The compact is one, if judiciously entered into, that renders the world alone worth living for. Man's earthly happiness, all other things being equal to his rights and expectations, rests on no higher pinnacle than in the union of hearts as well as bodies.

The reverse of the picture is foreign to my purpose. Marriage has its dangers, its disappointments, and its denials, and the mind and disposition are not more proof against the temptations of to-day than they were of yesterday.

It is an old idea, that when a man gets married he becomes settled, which implies that he is safe from the snares that surround single-blessedness. It is not always the case, nor are the chances of mortality invariably lessened by the change. I repeat, sick health, whether before or after wedlock, is not without its cause.

Herein do we behold the shoals and quicksands that lie under the apparently smooth surface of human life, and which so fearfully shipwreck the unwary voyager in the first half of what may be called " the grand tour."

The reader who has travelled thus far with me has now a moment's breathing-time, and the thought may suddenly occur to him —this is dangerous ground we are treading upon ; if he believe any one to be approaching, the book is thrust in the pocket, or perhaps thrown in the fire ; yet who can deny the truth of the charges herein made, and why all this monstrous fastidiousness ?

The same reader may not be so precise in his daily conduct in life—he may deal out a coarse joke, and consider the nearer it borders upon indelicacy the cleverer it is; yet what possibly comes home to him, through the companionship or possession of this little volume, he blushes to avow, and consequently would not, for his reputation's sake, it should turn state's evidence. The world has been making rapid strides in mental education—the schoolmaster is at home, not abroad, in every family ; but physical education (that of the body) is still very far behindhand. The dissemination of physiological truths should come from the medical profession, and although many professors have endeavored to popularize the laws of life, the one more immediately connected with the subject in question has been, comparatively speaking, entirely overlooked.

Books have been written on almost every complaint that has a name, and many have been printed to introduce a new disease scarcely known to any one else than the author ; volumes have appeared on diet, regimen, and medical hygiene of every degree ; but where is there a work to be found addressed to the growing youth who has his eyes and his ears open, and needs but the instructor to inform him of his error, which is written by any of our leading physicians and surgeons, whose character and reputation might add to its recommendation, on the subject of personal sensuality ?

The case of a disordered stomach is allowed to be a legitimate theme for a medical author to take up the cudgels for ; even the fruits of dissipation he is permitted to write upon, or to treat; but, alas! let him venture to moot the matter, in the remotest degree, touching the unfortunate propensity of the schoolboy, or the clerk, or the ploughboy, or the philosopher, and his character is gone for ever. And why is this? The jealousies of professional life, the morbid notions of what constitutes rigid respectability (WITHOUT USEFULNESS), and the rank uses made of human weaknesses by empirical rascality—all have helped to deter the respectable man from making the treatment of the consequences, and forewarning youth from the causes of this source of corruption, his especial province; and, therefore, wo be to him who courageously enters, as it were, on the forlorn hope of practice, to assist his fallen fellow man. It is not for me to speak of the part I have taken in the war against empiricism, or for the stand I have made, and fearlessly intend persisting in; but I have lived to receive—although, thank Heaven, not to feel—the bitterness of reproach. My integrity and moral propriety have been questioned by little and timid minds, or else denounced by journalists who live by slander, or *fee*-less rivals, who fatten only in their own conceit—" thanking Heaven that they are not as other men," (for which the public have reason to rejoice)—because I have identified my practice with the treatment of those diseases arising from the baser uses mankind surrenders his passions to—because I have boldly stood forward and defied the horde of quacks who have monopolized this department, while the qualified medical man, instead of doing his duty, listlessly looks on, and complains that government does not afford him that protection which he has in his own power to command; as though there should be no help to such; as though no wayward falterer from prudent living should be called back; as though the medical treatment, rather than the habit, was the more disgraceful pursuit; forgetting that " *the disgrace is in the crime, not the scaffold.*"

Before entering upon the more agreeable part of my task, of offering to the notice of the invalid, or haply new-converted reader the suggestions I have gathered together from my own and the experience of others, for general guidance, I will claim a page to comment upon what I have already presented. In drawing attention to the unhealthiness of free living and dissipation, and to the serious consequences of the addiction to licentious and other demoralizing practices, I need hardly say, that as I rail against their persistence, I am an advocate for their relinquishment, and the sooner that is effected the better. As a remedy for the former evils, and no less for the latter, it is evident that careful and prudent diet, temperate drinks, an observance of renovating regimen, and the adoption of an entire reformed habit of living, are indispensable The reading and thinking world is so alive to the importance and advantages of temperance, even to teetotalism, that a new work on the subject were almost superfluous ; but it is not so learned in the necessary restrictions and regulations of feeding, and in the exercises of the other appetites of the body, which many believe are given to us merely to be appeased, and that the comforts of life consist only of eating, drinking, and sleeping. This we shall presently inquire into.

As to the removal of those symptoms which do not give way to the new line of life, although the bard has bidden the healthy man "throw physic to the dogs," it must not be forgotten that

"For want of timely care,
Millions have died of medicable wounds,"

and therefore medical aid must not be despised. Much as I place my trust in diet and regimen, I bow with submission to the noble art of healing, and cling to it for succor.

On the subject in question a vast field appertains to it for consideration. Of course the first step taken to repair the ravages incurred must be by the immediate abandonment of the cause.

The idea of matrimony is ever uppermost in a man's mind. Physical training is not merely confined to the practice of medical men. Pedestrians, pugilists, jockeys, sportsmen, &c., have their codes of health, and by adopting them, attain the goal they aspire to ; and he who aims at wedlock, why should he not prepare for his duties ? It is a pity we have not some public examining office to determine a man's fitness, soundness, or eligibility for the step he is proposing to himself to take ; it would save many, many disappointments. The dowry of wealth covers a multitude of sins ; that of health however renders doubly sweet the compact.

CHAPTER II.

HOW TO LIVE, WHAT TO EAT, DRINK, AND AVOID.

"Fair golden age, when milk was th' only food,
And cradle of the infant world, the wood,
Rocked by the winds?"———

"Though I look old, yet I am strong and lusty,
For in my youth I never did apply
Hot and rebellious liquors to my blood,
Nor did not with unbashful forehead woo
The means of weakness and debility.
Therefore my age is as a lusty winter,
Frosty but kindly."

HAVING described the principal besetting propensities of early life, which it requires no very lengthened argument to prove lead to the break up of the healthiest constitution, it follows that what I have pointed out as productive of ill health should be avoided. I admit it is easier to preach than to practice, but if the assurance of one, who in his time has passed through the ordeals of excitement, of pains and pleasures, of the cares also and the anxieties of life, be worth the confession, I can pronounce that a little resolution, only it must be DETERMINED RESOLUTION, is all that is required. Nature will assuredly assist in the attempt. If a man find that by eating less, by avoiding stimulative drinks, by shunning bad habits, and by adopting a simple mode of living, he becomes better in health, and in reality feels the comfort of living free from uneasiness, and what is equally important, SLEEPING free from fright, he must indeed be a simpleton, if he can not control his appetites and keep to his new regulations. What can be more fearful than a night spent in restlessness, in tossing and twisting, in hideous dreams, with the necessity of turning out at a fixed hour in the morning, unrefreshed and with onerous duties to go through the day?

> "Not all a monarch's luxury the woes
> Can counterpoise, of that most wretched man
> Whose nights are shaken with the frantic fits:
> * * * * * * Whose delirious brain,
> Stung by the furies, works with poisoned thought,
> While pale and monstrous panting shocks the soul,
> And mangled consciousness bemoans itself:
> For ever torn, and chaos floating round."

What can be more depressing than to feel one's self incompetent for those very duties—to be harassed with, possibly, headache, with languor, with depression, with positive debility, with REAL NERVOUSNESS—to know that what we have to do MUST, or at least OUGHT to be done; that probably on its success depends our position in life; and yet, despite all our energies and convictions of its necessity, we find ourselves thoroughly incompetent to get through the day's work? Admitting all this, it is surely worth the experiment—and the success of it may be guarantied—of trying, or rather determining, to live according to the new regimen.

With this prosaical episode I enter on the considerations of "*How to live!*"—"*What to eat, drink, and avoid!*" and on the various other observances the invalid, however indisposed he may be to adopt, finds it imperative to submit to. These questions require for their solution some discussion on the following several points:—

The value and varieties of food; on quantity and quality; the importance and salubrity of fresh air; the necessity of different kinds of exercise; of rest, when and how much to be taken; of regimen and conduct generally, and the government of the passions. First, then, as to

Diet.

> "The watchful appetite was given,
> Daily with fresh materials to repair
> This unavoidable expense of life,
> This necessary waste of flesh and blood."

Without we eat and drink, we die! The provocative to do both rests with the appetite, which, in process of time, becomes a very uncertain guide; for the palate will often induce a desire and relish for that which is most mischievous and indigestible. The old sayings of "eat what you like," is now shunned by everybody of twenty years' experience. Still, without appetite, it is a very difficult affair to subsist—for the pleasure depends chiefly upon the relish. The relish may become, as has been stated, a vitiated one, but it is quite possible to make the stomach, by a little forbearance and practice, as enamored of what is wholesome and nutritious, as of that which is hurtful, and not concoctible. Food consists of solids and fluids, which severally have their different degrees of digestibility. It is proverbial that mutton is easier of digestion than beef—that fresh food is more readily dissolved in the stomach than salt—that it requires a pretty strong stomach to digest tough beefsteaks, and that he is a fortunate fellow who is not reminded now and then of having feasted on salmon twelve hours after, instead of four.

But there is a vast difference between the digestive powers of different individuals. It is impossible, therefore, to impose rules as regards specific quality alike for all. The grand principle in dietetics is for every person to judge for himself. When I am asked by an invalid what he may take, I inquire what best agrees with him. That fact ascertained, I bid him confine himself chiefly to the same. Most invalids of the class I have much to do with (nervous people) are great eaters; and although I do not allow them entirely to exercise their own judgment as to QUALITY, I invariably restrict them as to QUANTITY. Dyspeptics and others may rely upon it, that there is as much mischief done by QUANTITY as QUALITY.

It certainly is a very simple remedy for any one to diminish the quantity of his food, say one-third, or if necessary to one-half; but the proposal generally meets with opposition, under the idea that as strength can only be acquired from the food which is consumed, it follows, the more there be taken the greater will be the degree of strength got from it. Such a view is most erroneous, for it is only in proportion to that which is DIGESTED and AMALGAMATES KINDLY with the system that " goes to the good."

The delicate should feed carefully, not abundantly; it is not quantity which nourishes, but only that which assimilates.

    *   *   *   " While the vital fire
  Burns feebly, heap not the green fuel on,
  But prudently foment the wandering spark,
  With what the soonest feeds its kindred touch."

If a profusion be taken, it gives extra work to every part of the digestive economy—the stomach is longer employed, a greater supply of blood is required and furnished to the stomach, to assist in the creation of the stomachic secretions to aid in dissolving the food: chymical action, being always in proportion to the amount and dissimilarity of ingredients concerned, of course must be more violent in relation to the quantity, and hence there is greater uproar and confusion in the system to get through the task; consequently we have a quicker pulse, more excitement, and more exhaustion. Then follow flatulence, heaviness, and dulness, and sometimes sickness and pain. Let any person laboring under indigestion, or who may not feel comfortable after meals, just try and take one-third less of liquids as well as solids, and he will be agreeably surprised at the result. How common it is for a man to give himself now and then a holiday—to take rest as he calls it; but he only gives it to his legs and arms. On those occasions, having nothing else to do, he eats and drinks heartier than usual, and transfers his work to his stomach and digestive organs. He had better reverse the practice generally, as he would probably derive more benefit from resting his stomach than his body. I once saw a man eating a very hearty supper, and I remarked to him that his stomach would suffer for it. His reply was, "What did he care, so long as *he* didn't. He worked for his stomach, and his stomach must work for him;" forgetting, or not knowing, that he and his stomach were one—for upon the due performance of the stomach depends the health of the owner.

Another important feature is simplicity and singleness of living. Let each meal consist of as few articles as possible. Bread, meat, and one kind of vegetable, are better than a mixture of many others; but of course these restrictions are only necessary to persons of weak digestion, or who may be otherwise in poor health. The cold water curers and the homœopathists all build their faith, and achieve their success, by diet and regimen, rather than by the water and the physic. It is very vexing to find the absurd prejudices in families against simplicity of diet. The old joke is ever handy, if mutton be ordered, it being notoriously the most easily soluble and particularly nutritious of all kinds of animal food; yet the mistress, or the master, or some one, will exclaim that they are becoming so ashamed of mutton! mutton! that they expect they will not be able to look a sheep in the face. If mutton suit an invalid better than anything else, he has only to thank himself if he do not continue well, through substituting, for fashion's sake or the love of change, his favorite joint for that of veal, pork, or beef. Many invalids dare not make the change, but at their extreme peril.

To continue about quantity: the feelings must be studied, to arrive at a correct knowledge of when enough has been taken. By eating too fast we are apt to eat too much, for hunger requires time as well as quantity, to become appeased. In like manner, thirst may be quenched as effectually by half a pint of water as by a pint, provided it be drank slowly; and hence, owing to the rapid manner in which draughts are swallowed to allay drought, we are apt to drink too much. A good way to ascertain what quantity is most fitting, is to study the feelings after a meal, when that quantity which is digested the easiest, and produces the least discomfort, or, in fact, sensation, is the one to be selected.

Again : one meal should not too quickly follow another—four hours, at least, should intervene. Three meals a day are sufficient —a moderate breakfast, a good dinner, and a simple tea ; but when little and often are advised, a biscuit lunch or a cup of gruel for supper may be added. A very important observance is to eat slowly and to masticate thoroughly ; in fact, the food should be suited to the teeth. If the grinders have decayed, have them, if possible, replaced with artificial teeth. Never hurry through your meals, nor proceed to violent exercise immediately after. Never eat too much, nor too often. This is reiteration ; but a good hint can never be dinned in the ear sufficiently to those who may happen to read what is not congenial with their own way of thinking.

When you are puffed out after eating, it is a sure sign you have taken too much. Always leave off satisfied, but never filled to repletion.

> "Beyond the sense
> Of light refection, at the genial board
> Indulge not often, nor protract the feast
> To dull satiety.   *   *   *
> The stomach, urged beyond its active tone,
> Hardly to nutrimental chyle subdues
> The softest food."
> "Gross riot treasures up a wealthy fund
> Of plagues."

Ahernethy used to say, "Never put more in the oven than it will bake."

Never take what you know from experience disagrees with you.

Half an hour's rest should always precede and succeed a hearty dinner ; but sleeping after dinner, except it be a custom, and the diner be an elderly person, is decidedly bad. The dozer invariably wakes up feverish, with an increased pulse and a clammy mouth, and the process of digestion is by no means advanced. Agreeable and lively conversation carries the digestion on unknowingly ; whereas, the man who sleeps or watches, and broods over his symptoms, retards the process, and makes his meal indeed a weary one.

The dinner should be the substantial meal of the day. Meat breakfasts and meat suppers are injurious to persons who take but little exercise.

Never be dissatisfied because you can not eat and drink, and enjoy yourself, like other people. I admit it is extremely annoying to withstand the fragrance of savory food, and to defy being tempted to partake of it ; but the wisdom of resistance is a great triumph over appetite, and the avoidance of indigestion an excellent exchange for the brief delight of a delicious meal. If it unhappily be that you must, on pain of suffering, deny yourself many of the agreeables of this world, endure the mortification like a man, and, as the poet observes—

"Learn to suffer what you can not shun."

I do not intend in these hints to enter into a review of the relative advantages of animal food over a vegetable diet, or *vice versa*. My aim is merely to present every-day maxims that are the more universally applicable. Special cases require special diet, and there are some forms of illness wherein only a farinaceous diet is admissible; others where even water is only allowable; and every medical man is acquainted with cases where patients have subsisted on that element only from ten to twenty days. Temperance in diet, water for drink, and hard work for exercise, will save and prolong many a life, if the trial be but made. This fact is certain—the diet should be modified by the occupation of the party; the more bodily exercise, the freer and more generous may be the living; the lighter the exercise, and the more confining and sedentary the engagements, the simpler and blander must be the diet.

As a general rule, where meat is to be taken for dinner, mutton is to be preferred. It might be possibly imposing a difficulty to many of my readers, particularly those of the younger order, to urge a slice out of the thick part of the leg or the shoulder, and well done (roasted), as the best, or a cut out of the saddle or the haunch; because where the dining-table be at the hotel or eating-house, or perhaps the counting-house, much must depend upon the chance of what is provided for the public; but where those parts can not be obtained, the ordinary mutton-chop (cut thin), or from the neck—the "long chop"—and well broiled, is the best substitute. Where a man has to *study* living, he must keep under his desire for variety—when I say he must, I mean he had better. However palatable the joint of veal or the cutlet, or any savory preparation of it may be, it is sure to cause repentance.

Beef has the same objections. It unquestionably is a national and delicious meat, but only fit for a man in rough and prime health. Than cold roast beef, no joint is finer; it is a most tempting dish, and people generally eat too heartily of it. Boiled beef, both hot and cold, is a great luxury, but only suitable for the hardy and strong.

Meat pies are very objectionable for invalids. Pork, in all its forms, is very difficult of digestion with delicate persons, whether as bacon or salted pork, or whether as young or mature, roasted. Pork chops are notoriously night-wakers. Even invalids are not to be interdicted every kind of nourishment save mutton, but of all meats it suits the stomach the longest and the best. If there be no alternative than to eat beef, or veal, or pork, or else go without, why, supposing the would-be consumer is not an invalid of the severest class, let him take any of them, but certainly let him take less. Let him on no account lose his temper and pinch his feelings by angry abstinence altogether. If he know he shall suffer from tasting anything else than his favorite mutton, he is wise to leave the table. If he will accept invitations out, he must run the risk, if he desire to avoid being considered particular, and take what is set before him; but even then he can easily deceive his host or his neighbor by "cutting and playing" with what is put before him, without eating, and awaiting patiently till something is put upon the table that is suitable to his palate. I was once delighted at observing the philosophy of an elderly and agreeable gentleman who sat next to me at a public dinner, and who passed, seemingly tasting it as it was put before him, the soup, and fish, and game, and making his dinner off a slice of lamb, one small potato, one piece of bread, with a glass of table ale. During the whole evening he did not exceed two glasses of wine, and yet he was as convivial as the rest, and left one of the first. On my remarking to him his abstinence, he observed, "I have always lived as carefully all my life; it is true I have been compelled to it, and am enabled even now (being sixty-five years old) to mingle in society, and yet keep in good health. I will be bound to say I shall sleep better to-night than any one here present." And I have no doubt he did. Cautious eaters must expect a joke to be played upon them now and then. I was once asked by a merry friend to make one of a dinner-party, and consented only on being permitted to take what I chose, he knowing I was dieting myself. A large hot-water dish, with an immense cover over it, was placed with much ceremony in the centre of the table; in like due form it was removed, and from the mountain ran a mouse—beneath it was a solitary chop. The laugh aided digestion, and I enjoyed my dinner.

By-the-by, it is a golden maxim, always, if possible, to dine on good terms with oneself. A dinner does very little good if the eater be worried over his meal, or there be jarring and sparring about the inattention of servants, or the bad cooking. The litigation does not mend the matter, and each mouthful is swallowed with a chance of choking. Much might be said on this head, but it will answer as well to reflect upon it, and avoid the contention. But to proceed. The brain, tongue, heart, sweetbread, liver, kidneys, tripe, &c., of animals are severally nutritious, but vary in easiness of digestion.

Sweetbread, lightly and plainly cooked, forms a good meal for an invalid.

Tripe is easy of digestion, taking cautiously of its appendages, butter, onions, &c.

Rabbits, well boiled (but not covered with onion sauce), if young, may be eaten now and then; jugged hare, taking sparingly of the gravy, is occasionally allowable.

There is no objection to the occasional substitution of poultry, such as fowls and chickens, breast of turkey, &c. The breast of all birds is the most juicy and nutritious part, and that of the young more so than the old. Dr. Beaumont, however, considers chicken more difficult of digestion than beef, on account of the close texture of its flesh. He says it dissolves like gum—some invalids find it so; but I think the objection lies more when the bones are closely picked, and where the ligaments and tendons of the joints and muscles, together with the skin, fat, gizzard, &c., be consumed. Game is considered rather easy of digestion, especially venison, partridges, pheasants, and wild birds generally; but the chief objection to these dishes are the accompaniments, the sauces, the stuffing, the jellies, &c., AND THE QUANTITY.

Lamb is very excellent, and light of digestion, avoiding the fat, and usually suitable for invalids.

Curry is an occasionally permissible dish : rabbits, fowls, chops, cutlets, and many other small articles so served, vary the fare and rouse a torpid stomach to increased action ; but people must judge for themselves—with many curry is too stimulating, whilst with others it facilitates digestion, and allays morbid irritability.

There are innumerable make-shift dishes, which a clever cook and a good nurse know how to provide for the sick chamber, such as mild stews, broths, jellies,* and teas ; but, as I am writing more particularly for those who cannot, to the extent it might be wished, be choosers, and who have no nurses or cooks, I need not descend into particulars. If an invalid have the privilege of dining at a family table, or a hotel d'hôte, let him bear in mind the following remarks :—

Meat of nearly all kinds is generally in season, or can be ob-

* Calves'-feet jelly, likewise isinglass and hartshorn jellies, are good for invalids; but rich soups and hashes are indigestible, and provoke only thirst and flatulence.

tained all the year round, but it is most nourishing when what it feeds on IS IN SEASON, or is most plentiful. Grass is a better food than hay. Stall-fed oxen are fat and less wholesome than those of the leaner kind, who have their run in the meadows.

So it is with man.

It must be borne in mind, that the diet should be lighter in summer than in winter; this observation holds good to liquids as well as solids.

In summer, as the poet writes:—

> "The moist cool viands then and flowing cup
> From the fresh dairy virgin's lib'ral hand,
> Will save your head from harm, tho' round the world
> The dreaded fever rolls its wasteful fires."
> * * "Winter loves the gen'rous board,
> The meal more copious, and a warmer fare,
> And longs with old wood and old wine to cheer
> His quaking heart."

Eggs, lightly cooked, as when poached or boiled for three minutes, or baked (called at the Astor House, New York, the best hotel in the country, *Shirred Eggs*), are good. Fried eggs, as in pancakes, omelettes, &c., are bad. Some people find eggs nutritious taken RAW, in tea or coffee, or beaten up with wine. Egg-flip again has its advocates; every housekeeper knows its composition. For the beginner, it may be stated, that it is made by beating up an egg or two in hot ale, and flavoring the mixture with nutmeg, ginger, and some spirit, such as rum, gin, or brandy. Wo be to the dyspeptic who ventures upon it, although as a cordial to the weather-beaten man it is excellent.

Fish alone is at best but a sorry diet for a weak and delicate person; it is a good substitute occasionally when a whiting or haddock be selected, but, at best, it is obnoxious to a dyspeptic stomach. Melted butter and sauces should be particularly avoided.

The test of the goodness of white fish is, that it should be still whiter when boiled.

All fish should be eaten sparingly of.

Salmon, eels, herrings, pilchards, and sprats, abound in oil, and are enemies to digestion. Many diseases arise from eating fish, particularly if the fish be bad: fish is bad out of season.

Dried and salted fish are by no means to be recommended to weak stomachs.

Shell-fish are all, with the exception of the oyster, great disturbers of the stomach. Oysters are more digestible raw than when cooked, for roasting, scolloping, or stewing, only hardens them, besides occasioning them to be more indigestible, on account of the butter mixed in their preparation. They do not agree with all persons. A great object is to procure them fresh. An oyster-eater should learn when they are brought fresh to market, and only go to the best and noted houses for them.

I fear this will prove a most disagreeable chapter for an epicure, inasmuch as meat is recommended—and that meat MUTTON—as the chief substantial to live upon, and when people talk of falling sick upon it, when they know all other meats disagree with them, I have no objection to their practising still greater abstinence, and taking even mutton on alternate days, instead of consuming it daily. A fast of that kind is very advisable oftentimes for invalids, living in the meantime on bread and rice-puddings, and such like diet. I am principally commenting on the chief materials of the dinner-table—I will now speak of the appendages; and next, when I shall have presented a few more remarks on the quantity it is necessary a delicate person should limit himself to, I will conclude my "Guide" with a brief recapitulatory chapter, and the insertion of a set of gradatory diet tables for invalids generally.

Setting apart the *entrées* of the breakfast, dinner and tea meals, the diet of our country consists chiefly of tea, coffee, chocolate or cocoa, milk, sugar, bread, butter, meat, poultry and game, potatoes and other vegetables, cheese, and beer, with condiments. Abstracting from this list those which are not invariably suitable, and those which are prohibited by some medical men, we have only left bread, meat, and water, and so, in fact, the invalid has little choice remaining; still, of this, a man may regain health and thrive, and, moreover, enjoy himself.

It may, at first glance, appear next to an impossibility to a man who may have lived off a sumptuous table, that he shall, even with submission and satisfaction, dine off such humble fare—that he shall subsist on milk and water and bread, for breakfast and tea; and off bread, meat, and water, for dinner; and why not? The fact is, I have known hundreds do it, and they have been rewarded with a restoration to health for their pains and perseverance.

It does not exactly always follow that an imposition of this kind of fare is to hang over an invalid for the rest of his life, but it is the only way to secure a return to a somewhat more generous and cheerful mode of living.

Now, just for an instant, let THE free liver look over the following list of eatables, &c., that he is or has been accustomed to partake of during one or each day of his "joyous times," and he will observe, in *italics*, those *things* which have been, in all probability, wasted on him, or, in other words, that were unnecessary. On rising in the morning, a *glass of Congress water;* a smoker must have a *cigar.*

Breakfast—a *bowl* of coffee, whereas a small cup would do, or a *dish* of *strong tea,* a *plate of frizzled bacon, broiled ham, old meat, fowl,* or *some savory relish, hot buttered roll or toast,* bread and butter or dry toast being alone sufficient.

After breakfast—*a cigar or more, a dram, or a glass or two of ale.*

Dinner—*soup, fish, poultry,* joint, *various* vegetables, *savories, pastry, light wines,* possibly beer, *champagne, port, claret, soda water, and brandy;* the evening spent in a continuation with cigars. Now, mark, all that is merely necessary is the joint, vegetables, and beer.

I admit this man may hunt, may ride, may take plenty of exercise, and may enjoy himself in all the sports a young man with means may command : or he may lead a bustling life, may travel, and do most of these things with impunity ; then I have no fault to find with him, but so much of it is an outrage upon nature, and, sooner or later, he must give in, and then he cannot help regretting what he has caused. The majority of my patients have been men of this kind—men who have lived doubly fast, and are absolutely old at five-and-thirty.

Of Vegetables.

I shall not particularize the " vegetable kingdom" by an analysis of its orders, but merely take a view of the kitchen supply, or such as is most common to the dinner and dessert table. Bread comes under the denomination of a vegetable, and is best known as home-made, domestic, white and brown bread. We have varieties in the form of biscuit, pies, and puddings, made from the same material—flour. Of these I will first speak. NEW BREAD IS VERY UNWHOLESOME ; it should, by everybody, be eaten, after it is ONE DAY OLD. Invalids should have it toasted, and eat it only when cold, buttered or not, as may be. It must be recollected that bread is always imperfectly baked, the top and bottom being the only parts thoroughly done ; hence toasting completes the process. White bread has a tendency to constipate the bowels ; it is rendered more astringent by the alum the bakers mix with it. Brown bread, being made of coarser materials, that is, flour not so well pulverized and sifted, WORKS ITS WAY, and helps to preserve the bowels in a healthy and lax state. The best plan is to alternate their consumption, or take the brown bread for breakfast and tea, and the white for dinner; or reverse it if it be preferred.

Bread is usually fermented with *yeast,* or *leaven,* but of late years unfermented bread has commanded great consumption ; it is certainly more wholesome—more saving in the preparation, both as to time and money, and, what is well to know, less constipating and indigestible than fermented bread proves to be to many. The following is the best formula employed :—

To make white unfermented bread.—Take of flour* dressed or household, 3 lb. avoirdupois ; bicarbonate† of soda in powder, 9 drachms apothecaries' weight ; hydrochloric† (muriatic) acid, specific gravity 1.16, 11¼ fluid drachms ; water, about 25 fluid ounces.

To make brown unfermented bread.—Take of wheat meal‡, 3 lbs. avoirdupois ; bicarbonate of soda, in powder, 10 drachms,

---

* As suggested by Dr. Thomas Thompson, of Glasgow University, in a pamphlet published by Taylor and Walton.

† Never mind the hard names ; copy them and ask for the same at the druggists ; they are merely the common soda, by which the soda water powders are made, and the spirits of salts of commerce ; but it is better to obtain them by the modern names given to them. When more experienced in the manufacture of bread, it will be expedient to purchase greater quantities at a time. By the aid of a pair of scales and a set of apothecaries' weights, and also a four-ounce glass graduated measure, a large bowl, and pestle and mortar, all this specific trouble may be avoided. Cooks ought always to be provided with scales and measures ; and no guess work should be allowed in the making of puddings, bread, cakes, &c., &c.

‡ That is, *wheat well ground, but retaining the whole of the bran.* (Flour is much modified by what is called screening, or "officiously separating what nature has beneficially combined," and loses thereby about eighteen per cent. of its weight, *pollard or bran.*) They may be obtained separately, and mixed in proportion to that which shall be found best to agree. It is held that flour with the bran in it is more nutritious than without it ; in fact, it has been proved that a man can not long subsist alone on white bread (that is, bread made without the bran), but that he will survive and fatten on brown bread (bread containing the bran) and water ; it is therefore a popular error to suppose that the whiter the bread is, the better it is, for the whiteness is only produced by the alum the bakers put into it. *The quantity of alum or stuff used by bakers is frightful to learn ; " but they are constrained to employ it, because bread not whitened by its means, or which separates not easily, is rejected by their customers as inferior in quality—such is the effect of prejudice and ill-directed public opinion."* *Each quartern loaf contains from a tea to a tablespoonful of "stuff!"* which renders constipated bowels and bad digestion no longer a wonder to those who eat such a compound. Flour varies in quality and purity ; it is mixed with other grain, such as rye, oats, and barley, and it is sold under various names, as firsts, seconds, thirds : it is kept prepared at the bakers for all purposes, and when wanted to make brown bread, must be asked for under the name of "wheat meal." It can be regulated afterward, by diminishing or increasing the quantity of bran, according to the effects ; if not sufficiently laxative, have more bran added ; if otherwise, the reverse.

apothecaries' weight; hydrochloric (muriatic) acid, specific gravity 1.16, $12\frac{1}{2}$ fluid drachms; water about 28 fluid ounces.

The following are the instructions to the cook or housewife for carrying out the preceding directions: first mix the soda and flour well together—let the soda be well rubbed down in a mortar, and then scattered through a sieve over the flour, stirring them together in a large bowl. Mix the acid well with the water, which should be cold, or lukewarm, by the aid of a wooden spoon; then make dough, the thinner the better, in the usual manner, by mixing the flour and water as quickly as possible; divide it into loaves of convenient size, which had better be put into earthern pans, and put them immediately into a hot or quick oven. In about an hour and a half they will be sufficiently baked. The soda and acid used form, when mixed, common salt, but the process of their conversion, the effervescence, it is that expands the dough and answers the purpose of the yeast. If there be too much soda or acid, the bread will be correspondingly flavored, and, where lumpy, slightly discolored, but neither circumstance is of any moment.

A clever cook is a most valuable appendage in a family, and we need not wonder at hearing the enormous salaries some of them obtain, when we recollect how great is their responsibility in a large establishment. This form of bread admits of many of the usual modifications, such as the use of milk, and its conversion into puddings, cakes, and biscuits.

To make a good plain pudding, which may be rendered into plum, currant, suet, &c.—thus: Take of best flour, $1\frac{1}{2}$ lbs.; bicarbonate of soda, $\frac{1}{2}$ an ounce; hydrochloric acid, 5 fluid drachms; suet, $\frac{1}{4}$ lb.; ginger, $\frac{1}{4}$ drachm; water (more or less) 1 pint. Mix quickly, as before advised, and boil in a basin or bag.

To make Cakes.—Take of flour, $1\frac{1}{2}$ lbs.; bicarbonate of soda, $\frac{1}{2}$ an ounce; hydrochloric acid, 5 fluid drachms; sugar, $1\frac{1}{2}$ ounces; butter, $1\frac{1}{2}$ ounces; milk (more or less), $1\frac{1}{4}$ pints. Mix the flour and soda, then add the butter; then dissolve the sugar in the milk, and diffuse the acid by stirring it as before directed, with a wooden spoon; then mix the whole intimately, adding fruit at discretion, and divide the product into two or more portions for baking, which is best effected in flat earthen pans.

Bread, of course, is held to be the staff of life, and it is a great consideration how it can best be prepared. Few families have conveniences or time to make and bake their own, and it is no easy matter to persuade bakers that the plan as advised herein is the easiest, cheapest, and best, but it is really the case; and what is of equally great importance, it is more nourishing and wholesome, and to the dyspeptic invalid it is a most valuable corrective. Independently of its being very palatable, it keeps much longer than common bread, and does not so readily turn sour. However, the instructions are so simple and easy that the experiment is worth the attempt ; and were bakers generally to sell it, they would find the demand very quickly compensate them. The remarks I have offered of the superiority of brown bread over white as a laxative bear good, whether the bread be fermented or otherwise ; but the unfermented is much superior, as not only helping to keep the bowels in ordinary action, but as being positively more digestible, and instead of being productive of headache, acidity, irritability of stomach, flatulence, and other symptoms of dyspepsia, it is corrective and avertive of all these. In Liebig's views of the sustenance of life it will be learned that the several portions of our food go to form the various structures of our body ; such as meat and bread form especially the flesh, bones, and blood, of the human being ; portions of their composition go directly to support and nourish the bones ; vegetables, fat, and sugar, have a destination of their own Now, in the process of refining flour, of making it white and pure as it is called, the millers rob it of a very valuable quality, its saline ingredients, which ingredients are indispensable to the growth of bones and teeth, and are still required to keep them in a healthy condition. Hence do we attribute the weakly-formed bones, as evinced by the bent limbs and bad teeth of the children who have been fed chiefly on the finest wheaten flour, or bread which, as has been just now stated, is divested of its salts. The coarser food of the poor secures them stronger limbs and finer figures for their young children, where health in other respects is born with them. This is worth reflecting upon ; and since the conversion in my own person and family, and in those patients I have persuaded to follow my example, of consuming brown bread, or at least mingling it with white, and of late unfermented, I can bear testimony to its great utility, wholesomeness, economy, and agreeableness. It is suggested that mothers and nurses, when suckling their young charges, should consume brown bread—if unfermented so much the better ; for upon the same principle, just quoted, that the body derives its nourishment from food analogous only in its elements to itself, so it follows that, as the child is fed only from the parent or nurse, it must owe its preservation to the soundness of the source whence it exists.

In continuation of the subject on the varieties of the uses of flour, &c., hot rolls, fancy breads, rusks, and tops and bottoms, come under the denomination of fermented, while sea-biscuits constitute an exception. Cakes consist of bread flavored with butter, eggs, or lard, with raisins or currants. They are very indigestible for invalids and children. Country people have generally a slice of cake to offer as a complimentary refreshment, with a glass of home-made wine. A dyspeptic would have heartburn and acidity throughout the day, were he to accept such an invitation; but there are thousands of people who can do "that sort of thing" with impunity. Biscuits, when well and crisply baked, are wholesome and easy of digestion. Those containing caraway seeds, and whimsically called "Abernethy," are, in my opinion, as bad as pastry and sweets generally.

Pies and puddings are made of course, with flour and butter, or suet, and from a closer intermixture (apart from the properties of the butter), are less digestible than bread. Bread puddings, made with unbuttered slices of bread, form an excellent meal, or an adjunct to one.*

Macaroni or vermicelli, boiled in beef tea or broth, makes a nice soup. Macaroni or vermicelli† puddings are excellent. Rice puddings, baked and boiled, are both capital forms of diet. The former should be made and taken without butter, and with very little sugar.

Barley broth,‡ porridge, gruel, sago,‖ tapioca,§ rice powder, and

---

* *Bread Pudding.*—Grate half a pound of stale bread, pour over it a pint of hot milk, and leave the mixture to soak for an hour in a covered basin; then beat it up with the contents of two eggs. Put the whole into a covered basin, just large enough to hold it, which must be tied in a cloth and placed in boiling water for half an hour. It may be eaten with salt, sugar or sherry.

Panado.—Place some very thin slices or crumbs of bread in a sauce-pan, and add rather more water than will cover them. Boil until the bread becomes pulpy, then strain off the superfluous water, and beat up the bread until it becomes of the consistence of gruel; then add white sugar, and, when permitted, a little sherry wine. An agreeable aliment for the sick.

† Take two ounces of either, one pint of milk, four table-spoonfuls of cinnamon water; simmer till the maccaroni or vermicelli is tender; then add three yolks and one white of eggs, one ounce sugar, one drop oil of bitter almonds, glass of raisin wine in half pint of milk. Bake slowly.

‡ *To make Barley-Water.*—Take of pearl-barley two and a half ounces, wash them, and add half a pint of water; boil for a little while; throw this liquid away, and then add four pints of boiling water; boil down to two pints, and strain. Raisins, figs, tamarinds, and liquorice, are sometimes added to make a diet drink.

‖ *Sago Milk.*—Take of sago one ounce, water one pint; soak for an hour, pour off the water, and add one pint and a half of good milk, and boil until the sago is dissolved; then flavor with sugar, nutmeg, and wine.—*Sago Gruel.*—This is made by boiling the sago in water only; and it also may be flavored with lemon-juice, sugar, and spice.

§ *Tapioca Pudding.*—Take of tapioca two ounces, the yolks of two eggs, sugar half an ounce, milk one pint. Mix and bake.

other similar preparations are severally admirable articles of nourishment. Cookery wonderfully alters the taste, appearance, and quality of all farinaceous articles. The various farinaceous preparations make excellent jellies.

Much interesting information may be obtained by a morning visit, on a market-day, to the principal market. Vegetables will be seen there (supposing he make his tour through the seasons) the young bachelor had previously little or no idea of, and the bare enumeration in the following list will astonish. Take them as memory furnishes :—

Potatoes,	*Parsnips*,	Asparagus,
Peas,	Vegetable marrow,	Artichokes
Beans,	Seakale,	*Salads*,
Broad Beans,	*Greens*, and *Cabbages*,	*Lettuce*,
French Beans,	Turnep-tops,	*Radishes*,
Scarlet runners,	Spinach,	*Cucumbers*,
Turneps,	Brocoli,	*Endive*,
Carrots,	Brocoli sprouts,	Water-cresses,
Onions,	Cauliflower,	Tomatoes.

Potato,* the almost universal vegetable, has advocates and opponents for its adoption. Liebig says, a horse may be stuffed with potatoes, but life thus supported is a gradual starvation, although prisoners have been fed upon them with advantage. Baked potatoes are less nourishing than boiled, and mealy potatoes are more digestible than waxy. Potatoes in general engender flatulence. Onions lose their stimulating influence by boiling, and are then considered wholesome. The best onions are found in Mexico.

In the foregoing table, vegetables of less digestibility than others, or which require strong powers of digestion (for the two properties are not alike) are printed in *italics*. Allowances must be made for idiosyncrasies or peculiarities of constitution, it often happening that those soft, pulpy vegetables, which appear to melt in the mouth quickly, when swallowed produce acidity, or digest badly, and thereby alter the action of the stomach altogether, inducing wind, distension, and innumerable other sensations, which subside only as the acidity is neutralized or passed forward ; whereas, at other times, greens, turneps, and carrots, sit lightly on the stomach, and are disposed of without difficulty. Invalids, except they have reliance on their stomachic process, from their feelings, should not venture on them. Dr. Beaumont, whose opportunity

---

* As a substitute for the potato, during its scarcity, rice, served up plainly boiled, or "curried," is very nutritious and palatable.

of witnessing the digestive process going on in the stomach of a man who had an ulcerated opening in his abdomen is without parallel, thus supports the popular opinion about well masticating the food, selecting farinaceous food, and living sparingly of fluids:—

" 1. *That minuteness of division and tenderness of fibre* are the grand essentials for the easy digestion of butcher's meat. The different kinds of fish, fowl, and game, are found to vary in digestibility, chiefly in proportion as they approach to, or depart from, these two standard qualities.

" 2. *Farinaceous food,* such as gruel, rice, sago, and arrowroot, and likewise milk, are rapidly assimilated, and prove less stimulating to the system than animal food.

" 3. Most of the other kinds of vegetable substances are the slowest of all in undergoing digestion, and very frequently pass out of the stomach, and through the bowels, comparatively but little changed; and hence the uneasiness which their presence so often excites in the bowels. In a given bulk they contain less nutriment, and excite the system less, than any other kind of food.

' 4. Liquids are slow of digestion, and hence, in excess, are unfit for most dyspeptic persons."

A Few Remarks on Condiments.

Condiments are usually contrivances of man to goad a relish—to provoke an additional zest for our ordinary food. They doubtlessly succeed in their purpose, as the drover by his nail-pointed staff impels the poor tired ox to market; but the overwork is not unattended with mischief. Mustard, pepper, and salt, we become acquainted with from our earliest knowledge of cookery, and we look for them with meat as we do for bread and cheese to follow; but too much is worse than none. The pickles, sauces, oils, and et ceteras, are also acquirements that betoken man has not much confidence in his own appetital resources—"*chacun à son goût;*" at best they are but messes, and fortunate is he who, needing them, they agree with. Savory or kitchen herbs are merely ticklers of the taste; they do neither harm nor good—certainly not the latter, while they may disagree with a weak stomach.

I am not for excluding natural products, which are merely worked in, in legitimate boiling and roasting, such as spices and aromatics; I quarrel less with the sweets than the sours, and I find fault more with the compounds than the simples. I object to the stews and other recently-introduced French dishes, where the chief object appears to be more to fire the palate than to nourish and comfort the stomach. If my hints be not believed, I warrant a neglect of them will, sooner or later, bring converts to my way of thinking. Too much sugar is productive of dyspepsia. The effects of early addiction to sweets are manifested in children by their foul breaths and decayed teeth; and what should exempt adults from a corresponding consequence, more or less? Some tea-drinkers (*male* and female old ladies) will take three or four lumps of sugar with each cup, which, allowing from four to half a dozen cups, makes about two or three ounces of sugar, and this twice daily. The French drink of "*eau sucre*," I consider most objectionable. Coffee should be sparingly sweetened; the taste and flavor of the roasted berry is lost when oppressed with sugar.

Of Liquids.

Half, or more than half, of the aliment we consume is liquid; but there is no doubt, independently of that, we all drink too much. The drinks most familiar to us are—

Water,	Tea,	Broths,
Soda water,	Coffee,	Wines,
Congress water,	Cocoa,	Spirits,
Barley water,	Chocolate,	Porter,
Milk,	Toast and water,	Beer,
Gruel,	Soups,	Ales, &c.

An excellent chapter might be written on water; indeed there have been many, and at the present moment more fuss is made about it than since the flood. But I must confine myself to a summary of its virtues, and the objections to its universal substitution for every other drink. It is the mildest, most necessary, and salutary drink we have; it may, notwithstanding, be taken to excess, and those who dispute it will have reason to repent, if they venture on the experiment of taking it to the extent some enthusiastic hydropathists recommend. As a drink to allay thirst, no fluid or modification is equal to it, and it is best taken in its pure state.

If man were to confine himself to water alone as his common drink, he would NEVER NEED any other; but having been nurtured in the way of variety, and possessing also an HEREDITARY relish and want of modifications of it, we see, every day, individuals to whom water alone is a provocative to numerous uncomfortable, and indeed insupportable sensations; but, as a general remark, it assists the various processes of life best in its unadulterated state, and your real water-drinkers, not your converted tipplers, but original imbibers of the spring, are undoubtedly the most healthy and long-lived.

> "Nothing like simple element dilutes
> The food, or gives the chyle so soon to flow."

Water differs in qualities; it is hard and soft. The latter is most wholesome, but less agreeable. From water I will proceed to the mildest alteration of it, into tea, coffee, and the like. The effect of tea depends upon its quality and strength—strong green tea, or strong mixed tea, I consider as hurtful as fermented liquors. In point of nourishment there is none but what is derived from the addition of milk and sugar.*

Coffee is less objectionable, but it must be taken moderately; it is then nutritive and moderately stimulating. Cocoa, chocolate, and broma, are modifications for the tea or breakfast meal, and agree variously with different individuals; they are both preferable to tea as regards nutriment, but their effects must be watched. Milk† contains all the elements necessary for the nutrition and growth of the human body, but it does not suit every stomach. It is a very uncertain commodity in large cities, but it differs also in its quality as drawn from the cow, the milk of the morning and evening seldom corresponding—of course, it is much modified by the drink and the health of the animal. Gruel, barley water, and other farinaceous solutions, can not be too highly eulogized—they are the domestic physicians, and kindly ones too. A man may be brought from "death's door," and sent again into the world by gruel Omniverous as man may be, how powerless he becomes when ill!

---

* Tea, as a beverage to a person in health, is all very well, and forms a refreshing repast—it is also—where it agrees, a suitable one for the delicately healthy. In ordinary life, where tea disagrees, and produces flatulence and restlessness, at night, it is because it has been too strong, or preceded by too much wine, or that it has followed too closely a solid meal. Of course, what is luxury to one person may be poison to another, and we should all be guided by our own feelings. Dr. Johnson REVELLED IN TEA, CONSUMING FROM TEN TO TWELVE CUPS at a time; others, like him, find their intellect cleared by tea, while, *au contraire*, many are depressed and rendered highly nervous. Tea in the evening is rarely required after a late and good dinner—it only disturbs digestion; if thirst prevail and be insupportable, a glass of cold spring water is the best "tea" taken going to bed.

† Various drinks may be made with milk; such as whey, cream of tartar, alum, and tamarind whey. The milk may be acidulated with alum or cream of tartar in the proportion of 2 drachms to a pint of milk, which may or may not be diluted with water, and flavored at pleasure with sugar and nutmeg. For tamarind whey: 1 oz of tamarinds to a pint of milk boiled for ten minutes. Milk and Seine water forms a good nourishing drink for consumptive people.

He who could before demolish all before him when in rude health, now calls for his pap, and eats with his spoon !

Broths and soups have their relative virtues. Beef and mutton tea constitute the invalid's best friend.

Lastly come we to BEER, WINES and SPIRITS.

Poor malt and hops ! How delicious is a glass of mild country table ale—its pleasant bitter, its briskness, its BRUSQUE flavor—but where is it to be had? In London, there are thousands of ales, strong, high-colored, pale-colored, thick, thin, effervescing, deadly-lively, old and new, bitter, sweet, and sour. All of these have their admirers, but as articles of drink for the dyspeptic, except the mildest and purest forms—and then they must be free from the DOCTORING* and DRUGGING of the publicans—they must be avoided. The valetudinarian would derive much strength and nourishment from the occasional glass of good brewer's porter, but to the eternal disgrace of the trade—I mean the public trade —it is never vended pure ; admit, if you like, that there are exceptions; but is it not tantalizing, that where you meet with one good shop, you are disappointed at twenty others ? Palate a glass of beer or stout, and you taste the sugar, the liquorice, and the copperas : there can be no mistaking them ; and although we are told, "Well, they are all wholesome !" in the name of goodness, let each man be at liberty to take such only when he pleases. Why should they be foisted upon us with the porter ? If we must take copperas, let our doctors prescribe it for us, not the pot-boy ; and if liquorice and other sweets be indispensable, let us select the time and place for their consumption. The fashion now is in favor of pale ale—bitter ale ; it is all fudge to say they are, although they might be, the mere concoction of malt and hops. They (the better sorts, where in reality genuinely prepared) are certainly agreeable and good, and I admit wholesome, but there is nothing equal to CLEAN TABLE BEER. In my diet tables I prescribe them certainly, but I am only responsible for their efficacy providing they be good. Be it remembered again and again, I am only advising the sick. I trust I am liberal enough to look without envy or ill nature on the man who can dispose of a pint of genuine full-headed "Barclay and Perkins" at a draught; nor, if appetites and inclinations were regulated by public vote, would I hold up my

---

* Adulteration of beer is by cocculus indicus, a rank poison, forbidden on pain of 200*l.* penalty upon the brewer and 500*l.* upon the seller. Beer is also adulterated by quassia, grains of paradise, cayenne, &c.

BEER HEADING is composed of gum, vitriol, alum, and salt, to give a cauliflower head ! ! !

hand against any man enjoying himself as he pleases, so long as he conducts himself with propriety. But there are many people who, from habit, become extravagant beer and malt-liquor drinkers, not because they really want it, but because THEY THINK they can not do without it. The habit extends to both sexes; and, in the course of my professional experience, I have met many ladies who have declared that they could not dispense with a draught of porter or ale, for their lunch, for the world—that their dinner would be nothing without it, and they could not sleep a wink unless they had their usual quantity before going to bed. Such persons I have usually found irritable in health, annoyed with wind on the stomach, headache, constipation, &c., and yet all these symptoms have left as the malt liquor became dispensed with. Many quiet, and, as they consider themselves, temperate-living men, get in the same way, and accustom themselves to drink large quantities of beer. Laborers, pleasure-toilers, pedestrians, and others, can endure more fatigue in proportion to the less they drink of malt liquor. The quantity only stupifies them, makes them heavy and sleepy, and uncomfortable and weary before half their day's pursuit be over. A seasonable draught is all very well—a daily draught may do—the sick man may gain strength from it—it may be indispensable; but I am satisfied, as beer is to be got, the majority of invalids are better without. I am fond of a glass of good beer. I never drink it, because I can never get it. The patient I may advise it for may be more fortunate. Malt liquor, whether in the form of ale or porter, is less irritating than wine or spirits, and consequently less objectionable. MUCH of either is injurious. Porter is a very heavy drink, fattening, and constipating, and inductive of liver complaints and apoplexy. Ale in quantity acts on the skin and kidneys, and creates irritation in both. Of cider, perry, ginger beer, lemonade, &c., I say to dyspeptics, the less the better, but people may judge for themselves. The objections to soda water exist in the quantity and frequency of the draught; else, now and then, it is an agreeable drink.

Of Wines.

We have sweet home-made and foreign wines, effervescing, light and dry, and dry and strong wines:—thus those principally to be had in the shops, and usually to be found in private houses, are currant and gooseberry, ginger, and Malaga, with many others; next champagne, sparkling hock, Moselle, &c. The light and dry wines are Moselle, claret, hermitage, and those of Rhenish produce. The dry wines are port, sherry, Marsala, and Madeira. To pick from the preceding list those which are most ordinarily drunk, and especially which are in requisition by invalids, the number may be reduced to sherry, port, claret, and champagne. The excitement of a glass or two of port or sherry, or their brisker brother, Champagne, is most exhiliaating to a man in health, but to a delicate person, or one just recovering from illness, highly dangerous. The pulse will be raised from 20 to 50 beats by an injudicious glass of wine, and there are many people who had formerly been wine-drinkers, one bottle-men, say, from 30 to 50 years of age and upward, who dare not now touch a glass from its exciting tendency; therefore, in all those cases where wine is recommended to invalids, or where invalids venture to take it, it should be diluted and taken very sparingly. There are a variety of constitutions, and consequently a variety of effects. WINE, AT BEST IS BUT STIMULATIVE, NOT NUTRITIVE. It is apt, besides, to induce acidity of the stomach, to create fever, to disturb the urinary secretion, and to annoy the skin. Its effects, when indulged in to excess, are notorious: DRUNKENNESS, NERVOUSNESS and DEATH. The positive mischief of wine to persons in health is to be found only in its abuse.

"We curse not wine; the vile excess we blame."

I do not object to a glass of generous wine, or a bottle, if it suit a man; but who is better after a bottle? Will not half a pint, or say a pint, produce more lasting and comfortable feelings than a quart? and, if so, why should a man make himself ill? A man need not court misanthropism—he may now and then be gay, but excess is never justifiable.

I am so partial to wine, that I would take my *quantum* every day of my life if it agreed with me, but it suits me better to do without it. I avoid it not from niggardliness, but because I feel clearer, lighter; mouth and throat feel pleasanter; because I experience less fulness, less want of a continued aid to keep up the pleasurable feelings which one or two glasses produce; for in a drinking bout, the difficulty is to leave off—the succeeding glass is necessary to keep up the excitement of the last, to avert the dulness that invariably follows the decline of the hilarity. Wine also constipates—it interrupts digestion if taken at meal-time, or else hurries it, when the food is driven through the body but half dissolved. It is better suited for the active than sedentary, and the bustling than indolent man. To the deliciousness of the draught —the smack of the tongue—the exquisiteness of the swallow, or flavor, if it please better, for inelegant as these expressions may be, their truth can not be denied, I bow attentively; but still I do not take wine, or very rarely, and then only with great care and watchfulness—do not need it, nor do I feel the want of it; and I would advise my patients to be as cautious as I have become. I consider, although I never took wine to excess, nor have ever been but a temperate man, that I have added ten years of comfort and longevity to my existence, merely by abandoning it as a general practice; and if, in the course of conversation with any of my future patients or correspondents, I may be drawn into a confession of many other things seemingly harmless, because everybody adopts them, that I have given up, which I formerly took, and the relinquishment of the many customs I formerly practised, I have no doubt I shall make many proselytes from the ease with which these changes can be effected, and the good which surely follows their relinquishment. I am addressing dyspeptics and highly nervous invalids.

Of Spirituous Liquors.

Brandy, Rum, Whisky, Hollands, and Gin, and their Mixtures.

To denounce all these as poisons is excessively arrogant and dogmatic; yet many well-disposed persons have done so. I have in some of my earlier publications advised the same myself; and although my personal experience of their several effects does not authorize me to countenance the HABIT of using them, I would not discard them in a case of necessity; nor would I forbid the seasonable glass of grog to the fatigued and industrious fellow-adventurer in this hive of incessant work, or exclude its influence from the social table. Intemperance no one can recommend, but the good things of this world and those which are included in the present category are not designed for mischief. If man convert them into such, he has only himself to blame. The question at issue is as to their wholesomeness. They should be viewed as cordials, and taken for the same intentions as wine. For medicinal purposes they are incontestably useful, but they are quite out of characters as comforters for the depressed man. Their continual inhibition, night after night, either diluted or commingled together, is bad—is hurtful—is dangerous. The morning dram is most mischievous, and, persisted in, productive of diseases of the liver, kidneys, and absorbent and secretive system at large. Spirits should only be taken on certain occasions, to counteract specific conditions; as for instance, colds, fatigue, great depression, and other temporary disturbances. Employed medicinally, they form powerful adjuncts, at the command of the physician. Spirits are the preservers of many medicinal preparations, especially tinctures, which are usually prescribed as ADDENDA to infusions and decoctions, when ordered for the sick; and if admissible to the stomach in that form, there is no reason why the more agreeable cordials, added to warm water, instead of herbal or vegetable boilings, for the like purpose, should be excluded.

NOTE.—Alcohol is not nutritious. When swallowed it undergoes digestion, and commingles with the blood; but then, like all superfluities, it has to be thrown off. It is not detectible in the urine, fæces, or perspiration, but it is in the breath. Liebig says that it is given off by respiration, in the form of carbonic acid and water; that, in fact, it becomes oxydized in the lungs, and thereby heat is evolved. Grog or spirits always stimulate, and are taken with a view to generate warmth. That their habitual use on all occasions is bad there can be no doubt; but on the other hand, their essentiality in cases of exhaustion, or feeble health, or of extreme cold, is indisputable. Mr. Pereira (On Food and Diet) thus expresses himself against the above probable justification for dram-drinking. He says, "Though alcohol evolves heat in burning, it is an obnoxious fuel. Its volatility, and the facility with which it permeates membranes and tissues, enable it to be rapidly absorbed; and when it gets into the blood, it exerts a most injurious operation, before it is burnt in the lungs, on the brain and the liver; in which part it has been detected after death. Though, by its combustion heat is evolved, yet, under ordinary circumstances, there are other, better, safer, and less injurious combustibles to be burned in the vital lamp."

CHAPTER III.

RELATIVE DIGESTIBILITY OF DIFFERENT ARTICLES OF DIET.

Our journey in this life is beset with temptations, and the stomach, or rather palate, comes in for its share, and it is well an invalid (mind, these restrictions are not for persons in sound health) should know where mischief lurks. There is not "death in every pot," although the celebrated chymist, Accum, allows scarcely a single exception; but there are a vast many edibles and drinkables that are prohibitable to a person of feeble digestion, and otherwise nervous temperament. I will just, *en passant*, enumerate a few articles which should be, if not altogether avoided, at least very sparingly partaken of; and on the other hand a few which may be depended upon.

List of Articles of Diet, with the Time Required for their Digestion.

Articles.	How Dressed.	Time in digesting. H. M.	Articles.	How Dressed.	Time in digesting. H. M.
Rice	Boiled	1 0	Mutton	Broiled or boiled	3 0
Sago	—	1 45	*Veal	Broiled	4 0
Tapioca	—	2 0	*Ditto Cutlets	Fried	4 30
Barley	—	2 9	Fowls	Boiled	4 0
Milk	—	2 0	*Ducks	Roasted	4 0
*Ditto	Raw	2 15	*Butter	Melted	3 30
*Tripe	Boiled	1 0	*Cheese, Old Strong	Raw	3 30
Venison Steak	Broiled	1 35	*Soup, Beef, Vegetables, and Bread	Boiled	4 0
Turkey	Roasted or boiled	2 30			
*Goose	Roasted	2 30	*Soup, Bean	—	3 0
*Pig, Suckling	—	2 30	Ditto, Barley	—	1 30
Lamb	—	2 30	Ditto, Mutton	—	3 30
Chicken	—	2 45	Chicken Soup	—	3 0
*Eggs	Hard boiled	3 30	*Hashed Meat, and Vegetables	Warmed	2 30
Ditto	Soft	3 0			
*Ditto	Fried	3 30	*Sausages, Fresh	Boiled	3 20
*Custard	Baked	2 45	*Heart, Animal	Roasted	4 0
*Salmon	Boiled	1 30	*Beans	Boiled	2 30
Oysters	Raw	2 55	Bread	Baked	3 30
*Ditto	Stewed	2 30	Dumpling, Apple	Boiled	3 0
Beef	Roast	3 30	Apples	Raw	2 50
Beef Steak	Broiled	3 0	*Parsnips	Boiled	2 30
*Pork Steak	—	3 15	*Carrots	—	3 15
*Do., Fat and Lean	Roasted	5 15	*Turnips	—	3 30
*Do., recently salt'd	Boiled	4 30	Potatoes	—	3 30
Mutton	Roasted	3 15	*Cabbage	—	4 30

Those marked * should be avoided, or eaten very sparingly by the invalid, for it does not follow that that which is the more readily soluble is the most suitable to a morbidly sensitive stomach.

This list is founded upon experiments made on small quantities. Of course the more there be taken, the more time is required, on account of the suspension of the process of digestion, occasioned by the absolute irritation from the distension of the stomach. As far as my experience is concerned, I would rather the reader rely upon his own judgment for his guide than the time stated in the outer margin, as the time varies with the health and seasons, and with perfect or imperfect mastication.

Bringing my own observations to amend or augment the preceding catalogue, I find the following had generally better be AVOIDED by dyspeptics:—

Avoid.

Cream,	Marshed potatoes,	Sprats,
New bread,	Sausages,	Eels,
Hot rolls,	Stuffing of meats,	Cheese,
Fat bacon,	Do. of poultry and game,	Pastry in all its shapes,
Green tea,	Smoked beef,	Salads,
Buns,	Salt meat,	Raw vegetables,
Sweet Biscuit,	Peas, suet, &c.	Cucumbers,
Rich soups,	Marrow puddings,	Radishes,
Pork,	Fried fish,	Lettuces,
Beef,	Boiled salmon,	Nuts, walnuts,
Veal,	Mackerel,	Cocoa-nuts,
Ham,	Shrimp and other sauces,	Almonds and filberts.

A MAN IN HEALTH MAY PARTAKE OF EVERY ONE. THIS ARRAY OF "FORBIDDEN FRUIT" IS ONLY FOR "INVALIDS."

There may be many articles of diet omitted, besides new forms are continually being introduced, but the past observations and restrictions apply to those usually of ordinary consumption. Nor is the prohibition applicable to every individual case. I am quite aware that, when general advice is extended over so many pages, the attention of an invalid is very difficult to obtain, and that much time is required to gain over his adherence to what may not accord with his notions, but which, when enforced by the word of mouth from his medical man, he sets about in real earnest to accomplish.

Cooking.

It is somewhat presumptuous to trespass on the department of cookery, for housewives are generally the best judges as to the relative value of boiling and roasting. Whichever be the process selected, it should be carried out. Under-done meat is as injurious as over-done; and it is a popular error that states half-cooked meat to be more nourishing and digestible than well-done.

Baked meats are less wholesome than either boiled or roasted; they become "*soddened*," and have an "*oveny*" flavor. However, a great improvement has been effected in modern kitchen ranges, and the objection is becoming less tenable. The same remarks apply to the cooking of potatoes.

Frying is a process objectionable, chiefly on account of the butter employed, and the absorption of the fat into the meat.

A word or two upon fats—they are all slow of digestion. Dr. Beaumont says mutton suet takes four hours and a half to digest, and beef suet five hours.

Fat when swallowed becomes changed into oil by the warmth of the stomach, and floats on the surface of the food therein, until, by degrees, it becomes divided into myriads of little globules, as seen when water and oil are shaken up together, and then gradually mingles with the mass, and thus becomes digested. The fat of bacon is held by some writers on dietetics to be an exception, which is supposed to depend upon some change it undergoes in the curing; but my experience leads me to advise persons suffering under irritative dyspepsia to avoid it.

Read what Armstrong says:

> "The languid stomach curses e'en the pure
> Delicious fat, and all the race of oil,
> For more the oily aliments relax
> Its feeble tone. Th' irresoluble oil,
> So gentle late and blandishing, in floods
> Of rancid bile o'erflows. What tumults hence,
> What horrors rise, were nauseous to relate."

Quantity of Food.

The point settled, would, it appears, conclude the instruction an invalid can need. The secret of living certainly rests much on the quantity, but it involves several considerations, and the sick pupil must be a diligent observer.

Every person should regulate the quantity by his feelings. He ought to know when he has eaten enough. It is impossible to say with precision how much in general is requisite for every individual, for our appetite and capacities vary every day. Prisons and workhouses have their dietaries, but I trust my readers may be at least placed in the situation that they can command what they require, and have judgment sufficient to stop or go on, and take their meals when they please. This fact is beyond dispute, that more maladies are created by over-feeding than under-feeding, and it is also true that the majority of us consume more than there is really any occasion for. Every man in search of health should reflect for himself.

The better experiment is, if, on any given day, uncomfortable feelings ensue after dining, try the next time to satisfy yourself with one third less—if the same result follow, try the following day one half; and if diminishing the quantity still more do not succeed, try a day's fast. Dyspeptics accustomed to feed freely will find their health speedily improved by taking less; let their selection be judicious, eating slowly and carefully what they partake of. Above all, as I have remarked elsewhere, simplicity of living should be strictly observed, and the motto on every plate *should* be, "Temperance is true luxury."

"Nothing ever disagrees with me," will exclaim one; "I can digest anything—have a stomach like an ostrich." Ay, and well there are such, say those who subsist by them. It is true, thousands attain old age, and are gourmands or *bon vivants* to the end of the chapter. But what are they to the millions who can not and do not! Pick them out in a day's walk from one end of the town to the other, and what a motley group would they make!—what lean pates and paunch bellies would there be among them!

People now and then run into the opposite extreme, and endeavor to subsist on too little. The stomach requires only nourishment to *work* upon—hence bulk as well as nutriment is indispensable. To conclude this part of my inquiry of "when to leave off," having spoken but in vague terms of the exact how much should be taken, I will refer to the summary, and also to the diet tables, where the average specific quantity is given. Akin to quantity is the time we should take our repasts.

Time of Eating.

"To the rich man, when you are hungry," says the adage; "to the poor man, when you can." The latter advice may do for the needy, or the ever-at-work man, but regularity of feeding is of great assistance to a feeble stomach; a man, to be healthy, should keep time like a clock in all his hygienic duties, and, like many of the other daily functions of life, his appetite will, if thus encouraged, always attend him at the accustomed hour. Early breakfasts, midday dinners, and old-fashioned teas (at five o'clock, P. M.), with a biscuit at nine, are far preferable to the breakfast at ten, lunch at two, dinner at eight, and coffee at eleven. Our positions in life must modify these proceedings; there is nothing, however, like military regularity. One meal should never succeed another until the last is pretty fairly digested. Abernethy advised four hours between each. Eating little and often is a bad plan. Hence lunches, and buns, and biscuits, are severally injurious; they spoil the appetite for the more substantial meal, by calling into play—which a simple crust will do—the whole machinery of the domestic economy.

Snuffing and Smoking.

Medically speaking, they are both abominably unwholesome. They are delightful relaxations. Personally speaking (for I have been a snuffer and a smoker), I can bear witness to the great comfort and satisfaction I have derived from them. A cigar, during an evening stroll, is highly agreeable and companionable, but it is habit only which renders it necessary. It is pleasant, I admit (and ladies do likewise), to catch the whiff of a fine Havana on a frosty night, or an out-door walk. Nor do I object entering a bachelor's crib, where only real tobacco-smoking is going on—but a five minutes' stay therein is enough. To those whom smoking causes to spit, it is productive of great depression and considerable nervous irritability; to those who say they swallow their saliva, it is equally pernicious; to those who are insensible to secretion, it acts locally, and its influence is conveyed by the nervous extremities to the brain. It would appear ill-natured and cynical to forbid a solitary cigar; but as in this page I have only to do with its salutariness, I cannot speak in its favor. "I have never suffered from it," may say some one. Well and good; I do not forbid you taking one, but it surely can not be wholesome for those who do. Besides, what is agreeable it is very difficult to believe can be hurtful. Nevertheless it may be so; and smoking, in the majority of instances, I am convinced is so. What is the property of tobacco? —sedative, stupifying, creative of vomiting; and, if swallowed in the form of infusion, poisonous.

Let any man ask himself, after spitting and puffing, if he feel better for it; the reply generally is, "Oh, it is so soothing—it gives rise to such agreeable thoughts—it carries the mind back to the past—it makes a man comfortable even in his troubles. How happy every one appears with a cigar or a pipe in his mouth, from the lord to the basket-woman." A great deal of this may be true, but, on the other hand, the great smoker is generally shaky and nervous, and, like the drinker, never happy but when engaged in his favorite propensity. Of what use is he then to anybody, or even to himself? None. The little smoker, the occasional smoke breather, before he gets through his first, or give him credit for two or three, is left with a dry mouth and a nasty taste—a desire to drink: and although some will deny that smoking provokes drinking, except coffee or water, few can dispense with grog, ale, or wine. Other people it muddles, makes them swimmy, and very disagreeable to talk to. Many men smoke twenty or thirty cigars or pipes in a day, and a young town buck thinks it derogatory to his buckhood unless he can whiff away two or three. To say nothing of the nuisances of smoking, the habit, captivating and socializing as it may be held to be, is decidedly bad—very bad for delicate persons. As to *chewing*, it is an extensive habit. It is so beastly a one, that there is little fear of an invalid resorting to it. It is equally pernicious, nay, more so than smoking. Snuffing is sometimes used medicinally, and with great success. Light stimulative snuffs are useful in the affections of the head and eyes, and as a gentle refresher I have no objection to it; but real snuffing, where a man consumes half an ounce daily, and soils half a dozen pocket-handkerchiefs in the twenty-four hours—for those sort of snuffers awake purposely at night to take a pinch—is, I contend, very enervating, very depressing, except at the immediate moment, and extremely hurtful even to digestion; for, despite all the precaution, the snuff or its juice (bah!) will get down the gullet. Half a dozen pinches after dinner are allowable. Young men should particularly avoid becoming snuffers; a very short indulgence makes them look ten years older. These habits are very easy to acquire, and very difficult to leave off; but it is not, as some people say, dangerous to abandon them at the eleventh hour of your life. Mayhap such may not be necessary, but I have known people give up smoking and snuffing, which they had indulged in for years, at a moment's notice, and those people have been my patients, and they have soon found reason to thank me for the advice.

There is a joke I have heard of a great snuffer and smoker, who for some purpose or another got married, and, of course, out of deference to his wife, gave up both his favorite indulgences. He pined away, fretted, and went about like a shadow, soliciting and receiving the commiseration of his friends. Awhile afterward he was met by the narrator (who is supposed to be the retailer of the Joe Miller) in high glee, with his box in his hand and his cigar in his mouth. "Heyday! how is this?" exclaims his friend. "Oh! my lady smokes."—"But the box?"—"Oh! she snuffs." When ladies do these things I throw up my denunciation of the practice. The story is in defence of the habit, it being intended to show that some people, having accustomed themselves to bad propensities, can relinquish them only at the cost of tranquillity of mind, agreeableness of manner, and the sacrifice of health. The best hint I can give to a snuffer, to set the practice aside, is, to wear only a white handkerchief; that, beside locking up his snuff-box with a bold determination not to accept or take a pinch from anybody else, will cure him in a day. In a week he will forget he ever took snuff.

Late Hours.

To give a reason for every assertion in this little volume would render half a dozen keys necessary, which it is not my intention to do. I must therefore rely upon the common-sense nature of my assertions, and leave the reader, who, perceiving I state that " late hours are unwholesome" (to be understood idiomatically), naturally in his own mind says, " Why, what signifies when we sleep, so long as we get it?"—to solve the enigma by his experience. I assert the fact—LATE HOURS ARE UNWHOLESOME. "I thought so once, but now I know it."

"The body, by the toils
Of wakeful day exhausted and unstrung,
Weakly resists the night's unwholesome breath."

All nature sleeps at night, and why should not man? The great globe, and winds, and waves, move on, 'tis true, and the heart of man beats, and he himself respires, but these things are necessary to keep up the general order. The darkness of night is a simple proof that rest and sleep should be encouraged at that time. Of its necessity man is well aware; he could not, if he would, do without it. As IT IS, society could not well exist AS IT DOES, did it not encroach upon the hours set aside for repose; but AS IT WAS, our forefathers were wiser, and, rising with the lark, retired with the sun. A truce to this philosophizing. Invalids have little to do with balls, and routs, and evening parties, and persons who value their health will not turn night into day. Ten or eleven o'clock at night should never find delicate persons unprepared to go to bed. It is proverbial, because certified by actual knowledge, that the rest obtained in the early part of the night is more refreshing than that gotten in the morning. Rest is as essential as exercise. The vital energies become exhausted after their due performance, and require repose to regain their strength for the ensuing day. This is a physiological truth; and if that rest be denied, it becomes an infringement on a law of nature, and that is sure to bring down speedy vengeance. What are the feelings after being up all night! How doubly heavy is the sleep the next night! which, if not taken, the exhaustion becomes an illness. Evils are of two kinds—too much is as bad as too little, and he who retires early should rise early.

It becomes a disease where sleepiness prevails at a time when we ought to be getting up, instead of when going to bed; but one of the best remedies is to retire early, other things being attended to, and nature will do the rest.

Sleeping apartments ought always to be capacious, dry, and well-ventilated. The bed should not be too soft, and the bed-clothes should be as light as may be consistent with necessary warmth. The inordinate quantity of bed-covering sometimes used has a most relaxing tendency, by promoting excessive perspiration, and by rendering the body over-susceptible to external injurious impressions. Many persons are prone to the pernicious habit of closing the bed-curtains wholly around them, or else burying their heads under the clothes, and thus

"Cabined, cribbed, confined,"

they continue to breathe, during the greater portion of the night, the enclosed atmosphere vitiated by their own respiration; this is certainly a most unwholesome custom. If the head be well night-capped, no curtains are at all necessary.

The excellence of early rising, and its inspiring influence on both body and mind, have been themes for the poet's song and the sage's sermon. Early rising promotes cheerfulness of temper, opens up new capacities of enjoyment and channels of delight to which the sluggard must be insensible:—

> "The balmy breath of morn, the bracing air,
> The twittering songster's carol in the sky;
> The blooming pleasures that await without,
> To bless the wildly devious morning's walk."

It increases the sum of human existence, by stealing from indolence hours that would else be utterly wasted, and, better still, unquestionably conduces to longevity. All long-livers have been early risers, and—to descend from the poetry of the affair to mere matter of fact—it is remarked by the actuaries of life assurance companies (an exceedingly shrewd people in all that concerns matters of mortality) that early rising almost invariably leads to length of days. Now, as the habit of retiring to bed at late hours will hardly admit of early rising, THEREFORE the necessity of refraining from the one in order to secure the advantages of the other. From six to eight hours' sleep are generally held to be sufficient, and no doubt on the average are so. Our sleep is regulated much by the season. In winter, people lie longer, on account, they say, of its being too dark to get up before eight or nine. There is some plausibility in the reason, but the system in cold and dark weather is more prone to sleep than in light and sunny times. Invalids need generally plenty of bed rest, but then they should procure it by going early to bed. Persons addicted to late hours plead the parties they form members of as one excuse, and others insist that the evening or night are the only times they have for relaxation. This is all very reasonable for such so constituted, but, notwithstanding, late hours are unwholesome. Moon and star-gazing are bad for delicate persons. There is more health and strength to be found in the practice of seeing the sun rise, than in looking at it at any other part of the day. In fact, I know of no feeling equaling in delight that of basking or strolling about, unshaded by housetops or any other earthly canopy than the blue sky, in the first hours of the morning sun.

Of Exercise and Fresh Air.

Exercise and fresh air should be inseparable. They were born with us, but man built houses to shut out the air and lock himself in! Governments taxed the light, and it would appear, in proportion to our advance in civilization, we are setting at defiance the elements of health and longevity. We are absolutely beginning to be more careful of the dead than the living; we are concocting cemeteries out of town for our defunct relatives, but excluding air and space in our city habitable buildings for ourselves. It is true, here and there is an attempt to widen a street, but the new buildings are becoming approximated, instead of distanced. Man, in a state of nature, had to seek his food; to hunt for it; to scramble for it; and hence the difference between the stature and health of the wild Indian and the civilized man. Now, man need not stir from his couch for a meal. Look at the difference between the active mechanic, the artisan, even to the ill-fed Irish laborer, and compare him to the confined clerk, the shopman, or the indefatigable stay-at-home of a master, and the evidence of one's eyesight must proclaim in favor of the former—must proclaim that exercise, with moderate sustenance, contributes more to health than high feeding, indolence, and every other enjoyment.

A pensive man, absorbed in his own thoughts, looking from his own window, little dreams of what a tissue of moving atoms he is composed. His blood is travelling onward perpetually; fluids are being deposited on surfaces and again absorbed; his heart is continually beating; his lungs expanding and contracting; and even the viscera have their folds in incessant motion. His very structure adapts him for locomotion; and the composite movements alluded to are mainly dependant upon that locomotion for their healthy persistence, and yet, like a tired horse, how loath he is to stir. What a subject to dilate upon! It is a science in itself. There is nothing still in nature but man (comparatively), and he is called restless. How many of our diseases are attributable to inactivity and confinement.

That exercise and fresh air are essential and salutary—that they are invigorative—that they afford strength and power—that they beget and preserve health—who can deny? That, on the contrary, indolence and confinement sicken the heart, sear the mind, impoverish the body, and shorten life, there can not be a single doubt. What then, is it that makes men prefer the latter, or, if not prefer it, yield to it? Necessity? In some degree it is, but in a greater degree it is either indolence or ignorance, perhaps both. The moment a man gets comfort around him, he prefers his ease, his " OTIUM CUM DIGNITATE," and there is a spirit of misappropriation present in young men's minds that leads them to seek relaxation of another, rather than a healthier kind. The theatres, the taverns, the town rendezvous, &c., have attractions more powerful than the morning stroll in the high roads and the fields, and if the one be indulged in, the other cannot be availed of. Exercise and fresh air are essential for the due performance of every function of life. By their aid digestion is effected, the proper action of the bowels and skin sustained, sleep secured, a clear head acquired, and life preserved.

"Well, Mr. Orator, granted all this; but pray how are they to be obtained? How am I, a banker's or merchant's clerk, engaged from ten till four, or nine till eight, as some of us are, to get them? Where's the liberty to come from?" "How am I," asks another, " a hosier's assistant, shut up from eight to eight?—a druggist's shopman, from sunrise till midnight?—a publican's barman or a butcher's apprentice (both as much entitled to health as a gentleman of a thousand a year), never allowed out—how are we to get them?" Ay, there's the rub. You must fight your own battles. The town is astir and in your favor. I can but little help you; my province is to tell you you ought to have air and exercise—yours is to obtain them. "Where there's a will there's a way." Young men not compelled to sleep at their employers' warehouses, or business houses, should endeavor to get lodgings out of town, and should walk to and fro. Every half or whole holyday that can be obtained should be spent abroad. The stripling or youth, bound to the desk or counter, and who perhaps sleeps under it, should rise betimes in the morning, and take a stroll round the nearest open space he may reside most contiguously to—the bridges, the quays, the high roads, the parks, or the fields, if his master will allow him and can spare him. We can not all be the choosers of our time. I, for instance, although I have been five-and-twenty years at it, am still the servant of the public, and likely, mayhap, to be (at least I hope so) for some years to come. I can not, but at my peril, absent myself from my domicil at my appointed hours; and it provokes a sort of melancholy reflection to think that every evening, night after night, summer and winter, from seven to nine (Sundays excepted), I must always be at my post. I sometimes yearn for an evening stroll across the fields, a country ride, a steamboat trip, or a winter evening's amusement, apart from professional business, but it is in vain. Necessity has no law, it's ONLY compulsory, and I must abide by it. However I contrive, notwithstanding, to obtain my relaxation at other times. I am making this article very egotistical, but in my love for fresh air, and my conviction of the value of exercise, I consider my own feelings a tolerably correct standard of other people's, and what I am enabled to obtain, perhaps at some cost (for it is likely, were I to be at home all day, I might increase my gains), others might do likewise. The healthfulness of a morning's walk before breakfast has often been questioned. I can personally speak in favor of it. *I can never suffer* (voluntarily) *a fine morning to pass, winter or summer, without a two or three miles' walk, or half a dozen miles' ride or drive, and I meet many other pedestrians, equestrians, &c., on the same errand.* The reason why the morning trip is not always congenial, is very frequently owing to the late hour of retiring the previous night; and where the objection is that it produces qualmish sensations on an empty stomach, the better way is to eat a biscuit before starting.

Now, with regard to exercise on a more extended scale. To those who have it in their power to avail themselves of it at all times, to those blessed with equipages, they have, indeed, a powerful means of collecting health at every jaunt.

Of all kinds of exercise, walking is the most natural—horse-riding the most delightful, and also the most advantageous, inasmuch as a greater distance can be got over—a greater variety of air be respired, at the cost of positively more exercise, and less fatigue; besides, the country can be reached, which is no easy matter to accomplish on foot. Your horse should be a sure-footed one—over whose neck you can trust the reins to hang—one who will trot, walk, or canter. If carriage-riding be preferred, or be more convenient, or the only sort of conveyance attainable, pray let it be an open one, else riding for the benefit of the air is ridiculous. In travelling, always select the outside—people only take colds by fearing them; an umbrella, or a great coat, will always keep off the wet. The time of taking exercise should be between meals, neither immediately upon, nor just before one. The amount must rest on the time that can be spared—distance is less an object than time. A valetudinarian should be out in the open air as many hours as possible during the day, and the man in health, to keep so, should, at least, be on foot or in the stirrups three or four hours daily. The feeble plead inability to get about, and the indolent will justly tell you, exercise doth not agree with them; but the habit of inactivity once broken, it is astonishing how luxurious exercise becomes. Weak parts become strong, and health and strength are acquired every day.

By exercise abroad, not only do diseases of the body give way, but also those of the mind. A fit of blue-devils is invariably cured by a ride on horseback—there are so many things to engage the attention when seated on a cheerful, sprightly pony, and passing by different objects, that new currents of thought are driven through the mind, despite the greatest determination to be sad. Independently, when mounted, of the benefits arising from motion—from mental employment, and the necessary attention to keep one's seat, the lungs are having a feast of their daintiest relish, as we find ourselves carried " over the hills and far away;" the blood becomes purified, and whizzes to its uttermost confines; and the rider, in a short time, feels in reality a new man. It is something to fancy we have no life within us, but it is another to know we have life under us. Exercise cures constipation, corpulency, nervousness, and all forms of indigestion. A simple evidence of the importance of exercise is to be found in the majority who are busily engaged during the week, and who take what they call rest on Sunday—that is to say, who do not go out all that day. There are many who neither dress nor shave on a Sunday, but eat, and drink, and sleep. Without appealing to any one in particular, for they include rich as well as poor, I may ask, at least, whether the Sunday indolence does not make the Monday a less agreeable day than the Saturday? The extra feeding has a good deal to do with it, but the want of the usual excitement of business (the exercise of the mind), and the usual bustling about (the exercise of the body), are not uninfluential. Day promenading is more beneficial than walking about in the night air. In wet weather, when out-door exercise is scarcely available, pacing the passage with windows open is a good substitute. A man may walk many miles in his own chamber. Gymnastic pastimes are recommendable—the use of the dumb-bells—skipping—games of ball—battledore and shuttlecock—in fact, any pursuit that keeps the body active. Friction with the flesh-brush is no bad imitation of exercise.

> "The garden yields
> A soft amusement, a humane delight,
> To raise the insipid nature of the ground."

Persons engaged in sedentary pursuits—the LITERATEUR, the clerk, and professional man, need not fix themselves to their seats throughout the day.

> "To stand and sit by turns,
> As nature prompts, is best, but o'er your leaves
> To lean for ever, cramps the vital parts,
> And robs the fine machinery of its play."

There are many contrivances now sold under the name of "*Easels*," to fix a stand for books, to chairs, tables, &c., by which the change of position is less irksome than where you have to hold, perhaps, a candle in one hand and your manuscript in the other.

He, again, whose occupation binds him to his books, the student or the sage, if he cannot well pace his closet, book in hand, should read aloud; independently of having what he reads more indelibly impressed upon his mind, his lungs gain tone, and his respiration is rendered easier and stronger. Besides, it is excellent practice;—

> "The chest, so exercised, improves its strength."

Exercise, while it gives energy to the mind and body, provokes the exhaustion to insure repose.

I have spoken of air in combination with exercise; fresh air, under any circumstances, is of vast importance. How many pant for it, and how delicious to a citizen is its fragrance.

> "Ye who amid the feverish world would wear
> A body free from pain, of cares a mind,
> Fly the rank city. . . . .
> . . . . The rural wilds
> Invite, the mountains call you, and the vales,
> The woods, the streams, and each ambrosial breeze,
> That fans the ever-undulating sky:
> A kindly sky, whose fostering power regales
> Man, beast, and all the vegetable reign."

What has not fresh air, or, as it is called, when quitting the crowded city, change of air, effected! How many has it not snatched from the jaws of death! How many has it not saved from the tedious pilgrimage of sickness, and spared from desolate loneliness! The apparently consumptive, the melancholy hypochondriac, and the waning and harassed dyspeptic, has it restored to former lifefulness and joy. The first gush revives the expiring breath. Bed-ridden invalids have been known to rise and walk the day following a removal into the country. Apart from local peculiarities and advantages, fresh air is in every instance useful. These are not mere rhapsodies, but eulogies which the recollections and daily experience of all can substantiate.

The present facilities for obtaining fresh air far exceed those of former times, indeed even only of ten years back ; and he must be regardless or very apathetic of his own health, who does not now and then avail of them to get a sniff of the country. The railroads, omnibuses, and steamboats, are boons, despite their monopolies, nuisances, and dangers, that while they have their annoyances, which we every day are holding up to censure, we ought to be charitable toward, and trust to time for improvements.

The best time for riding for health, enjoyment of the country, and for the purposes of exercise, is certainly in the morning before breakfast, when the season will admit of it ; say from six till eight or nine in the morning. Despite the objections to getting up early, the horror which some people have of it, and the many real hindrances, let the experiment be but made, and the temptation to repeat it will be very strong ; besides the quietude, freedom from annoyances on the roads, the air is so much fresher, purer, and more delightful than at any other time of the day. Pray try it! If starting out upon an empty stomach destroy the pleasure, take a small cup of coffee and a biscuit or rusk, or biscuit or rusk only, or a crust of bread.

Where other times in the day can be spared, take the two or three hours before dinner, or else the evening also, or all three ; but the valetudinarian can not be too much out in the open air : it is the natural breathing-place for every one.

Every hour in the day has its charms : the rising and setting of the sun will find worshippers, but extremes may be avoided. It is not necessary to get up at three in the morning, or wait till the dew falls in the evening, or to melt in the noonday sun ; but from five or six till nine, or from nine until eleven, A. M., from three till six, or six till nine again, P. M., are remunerative ; but of course, weather, season, and conveniences must be studied.

CHAPTER IV.

ON THE PASSIONS.

"'Tis the great art of life, to manage well
The restless mind."

THE most powerful emotions are anger and despair. Scarcely a day passes but we hear of the fatal consequences of giving way to both. The intermediate feelings, the gradatory progress from simple irascibility of temper to ungovernable fury, and from mental depression to the depths of imaginative misery, that we see exhibited around us, swell out the list of human grievances that beset our travels through life. It is not to be expected that man can so tamely view aggressions, or so firmly withstand misfortunes, as to pass onward, unscathed by one or the other; but there is a certain amount of philosophy, necessary to meet misfortunes, which, if we do not possess, we ought to endeavor to acquire, else, like the reed, we should be shaken by every wind.

"But as the power of choosing is denied
To half mankind,"

it is the duty of all to fit their temper to their circumstances, and not suffer trifles to annoy them—to vex or depress them. The mind can be cultivated to withstand the shocks of the disasters common to the world, and also to resignation for those which can not be averted.

"Serene and master of yourself, prepare
For what may come, and leave the rest to Heaven."

The leading passion in human nature is irritability of temper; it is the source of nearly all our own discomfort, and that of those around us, and yet how easy it is, with a rational mind, to conquer and subdue it. If it led to any good result it might prove a healthy ebullition, but as it merely excites the brain, and to no good purpose, and seldom gains the end which reasoning might not accomplish, it is a waste of bitterness and even time, at the cost oftentimes of serious personal disturbance. Women have been thrown into hysterics, that have led to epilepsy and death, by indulgence in angry disputations: and men have sacrificed friendships, broken the peace of homes, and scattered desolation among their dependants and followers :—

> " For one irrevocable word,
> Perhaps that meant no harm, you lose a friend;
> Or in the war of words, your hasty hand
> Performs a deed to haunt you to the grave."

And such is life. It has been thought next to—nay, it has been believed to be—an absolute impossibility to govern the temper; that as everything in these days depends upon organization, if we are organized to be murderers, the crime must follow, and he only is virtuous who is happily abundantly possessed of the moral faculties. The young "LIMB," the SCOLD, the TERMAGANT, the violent and hasty man, exclaims, " I can't help it," and on viewing the destruction that may have been effected, cries out, " I don't care." This is a most fallacious notion. Phrenologists, at the same time that they admit that organization influences our conduct, know full well and insist upon it, that our conduct, or rather education, influences our organization, and that organization may be cultivated; that bumps, as they are styled, can be encouraged and depressed, and their contents called into action or subdued; and therefore, if phrenology mean anything, it means that viciousness and virtue depend entirely upon cultivation, and that such folly OUGHT to be helped and OUGHT to be cared for. "Bring up a child in the way he should go, and when he is old he will not depart from it." But it is even possible to alter habits of a later growth; and as, in the regulation of health, man must "chalk out" his own conduct to secure it; so in the control of his wayward feelings, he must bestow a little attention in the study how to do it. So much for the morbid excitement of passionate phrensy.

Even in a selfish point of view, irascibility of temper ought at all times to be checked. The flushed forehead, the blanched lips, the swelling throat, the fierceness of eye, and the towering voice displayed in an ordinary fit of anger, are pretty sufficient indications of the tumult within and the spirit without. There are few of us so irritable that we cannot repress these ebullitions of temper IF WE LIKE, at least to a very considerable extent; and, as it is confessedly very difficult to stay the torrent when in full flow, it behooves us to determine, in those seasons when reason is sufficiently cool to counsel correctly, to place that salutary restraint upon our propensities to passion and acerbities of temper, WHICH NEVER DO ANY GOOD TO OTHERS, and are sure to prove injurious to ourselves.

A calm, serene, and cheerful mind MAY BE SECURED BY CULTIVATION; even persons of a naturally fretful, peevish, irascible temperament will be astonished to find how comparatively easy it is to control and regulate their humors, if they will but *resolutely determine to bring them under domination.*

It is not my province here to dilate upon, nor to fathom the operations of the mind upon the body, arising from

> "*Anxious study, discontent, and care,*
> *Love without hope,*
> *And fear and jealousy.*"

but it is imperative I should not pass over the antagonist to the one I have chiefly considered, and that is DESPAIR. Despair is but the nurtured offspring of gloom and depression: it is a growing thorn in the heart of man—it makes him

> "*Sick in lethargy before his time.*"

Melancholy or mental nervousness, as it may be called, is generally the handmaid to the sick couch; not always so, but more particularly upon the complaints these pages are consumed in depicting. Here the faint-hearted man, unlike his angry brother, weeps in his regret, rather than gloats in his revenge; neither more nor less does he demand our sympathy. The two conditions are the saddest of suffering humanity. Like anger, it occasionally attains its climax, and it then may be called "human weakness" —nay, "folly." A *man* may *feel* his *sorrows* like a *man*, but, to antedate the quotation, he should also *bear* them like a *man*. In these fits of extremes the senses may be held to be at fault, and mayhap they may be, but in all errors there must be wrong somewhere; the question is, cannot the feelings of depression—the abandonment to grief—the absolute despair, which often ends in self-annihilation—be corrected? can not it be checked? can it not be removed? My belief is, it can.* It is not merely to be

---

* It is a little digression, but I cannot help recommending the reader, if this part of our subject come home personally, to procure my little book, called "How to be Happy." I have received assurances from many that the reading of it has rendered them so, by provoking a mode of viewing things in a manner till then they but dreamt of, but never carried out practically. I have quoted therein an instance of a man who appeared, and was always contented; and on being asked how it so happened, replied, "*I never suffer anything to vex me.*" It has been my aim, in the publication referred to, to encourage the imitation of such a philosopher, and to show how it may, has and can be done.

achieved, I admit, by resolution; for the resolution, unsustained by a removal of the cause, doubles upon itself and becomes as naught; but where the cause is known to be irremediable, the next wisest part to play, is to put up with it, for desponding will not remove it. We must remember the fable of Hercules and the wagoner. The god rebuked the lout for his tears, and bid him whip his team, and put his own shoulder to the wheel. He did so, and soon got out of the rut. Richelieu exclaimed to a hopeless adventurer, "Despair should not be found in a young man's vocabulary." Whatever the dilemma we may be in, our first effort should be directed to its removal. The more we fret, the further we are off. In nearly all nervous affections there is a strong tendency to depression of spirits; it is part of the malady, it may be as much the occasion of it as the consequence; and in the attempt to cure the disease, likewise, must our efforts be carried to the cause as well as to the symptoms. A morbid dulness is even soothing to some minds; and so easily are impressions caught up, that set but the train in motion, and the thought is established.

The melancholy man knows no comfort but in doling out his griefs; he ponders over his imaginative distresses and delights in his woes. Night affords no respite to his sufferings; for sleep—

> "Like the world, his visit only pays
> Where fortune smiles; the wretched he forsakes.
> Swift on his downy pinions flies from wo,
> And lights on lids unsullied with a tear."

ALL ADVERSITY FINDS EASE IN COMPLAINING, AND 'TIS A SOLACE TO RELATE IT.

Seneca adviseth—"To get a trusty friend, to whom we may freely and sincerely pour out our secrets. Nothing so delighteth and easeth the mind as when we have a prepared bosom, to which our secrets may descend, of whose conscience we are assured as of our own, whose speech may ease our succorless estate, counsel relieve, mirth expel our mourning, and whose very sight may be acceptable unto us."

Comminius told the duke of Burgundy, who was distressed in mind, "First pray to God, and lay thyself open to him, and then to some special friend, whom we hold most dear, to tell all our grievances to him. Nothing so forcible to strengthen, recreate, and heal the wounded soul of a miserable man."

It is of no use bottling up grief—out with it. "Give sorrow words." A good flood of tears oftentimes assuages the severest trouble; but when your feelings have had their vent, set immediately about repairing the breach in your mind's tranquillity.

Pondering on the one continual subject is like the gnat buzzing round the candle, which induces the same result—personal destruction.

It shows a bad spirit to rebuke a nervous person; it is an ill-natured feeling that would do it; but the endeavor to rally, to decoy, to entice away the phantom, is justifiable; a cheerful companion is indispensable. How catching is a smile, a laugh, or any exhibition of hilarity! it runs like an electric shock through a whole assembly. Who, also, can help sharing the sorrow with the mourner? and a pensive, thoughtful, and depressed attendant upon a subject of this class is like heaping coal upon coal, and smothering what little spark of life may be in the grate.

Of all things in the world to cure depression of spirits, occupation is the most powerfully effective; no matter the pursuit, anything is better than giving way to the one thought. I have known nervous persons recover through undertaking to read Scott's novels; another from the study of music, French, &c. In fact the resources are innumerable, if a ready and really interested person can be found to suggest them.

Persuasion, reason, and ridicule, have all been tried to rouse a nervous and desponding man from his gloom. The dark hour is upon him, and he will not be comforted. And yet how remarkable it is, the turn of his thought is occasioned oftentimes by the veriest accident—a gleam of sunshine, a fine day, an apt joke, or tidings of good news, will enliven him and give him many cheerful hours. The dram-bottle, which many fly to, is a poor resource. The best remedy I know of is—

RESOLUTION: the prescription should be compounded by a kind, PATIENT, and considerate friend; its ingredients are a rational view of the case, a remonstrance against the absurdity of flinching from the destiny of one's common nature, an exposition of the utter uselessness of repining for what perhaps can not be altered, and sufficient firmness to insist on an effort being made to throw off the hydra, and again to "MINGLE WITH THE BUSTLING CROWD" and cheerful haunts of man.

Should the reader be perusing his own case, I trust this book will not be read in vain. He will find in other pages than this which faces him the groundwork of his own cure, else what I have written on the great principles of life—viz., diet, air, and exercise —will be, indeed, written to little purpose.

An author should not bespatter his own praise, but he may con-

rive at it by all fair means. I have no fear of not finding an advocate to bepraise the means I would employ in my pamphlet, entitled "How to be Happy." If it concern you, my friend, pray procure it.

I had nearly omitted mention of a very fertile source of nervous derangement; and although, while enumerating late hours, it must have been supposed I included the various midnight pastimes, besides smoking, drinking, and sensual corruptions, still not having specified them, they may by some be considered merely as forgiveable faults. The especial one I have in view, and which I may not inaptly introduce here, is

Morbid Excitement.

What harm is there in a rubber—a quiet rubber? None! And one cannot help now and then prolonging the break-up to finish the last game—no objection. Billiards also, like cards, can only be well played at night; and if these two gentlemanly and social amusements are to be forbidden, because some hard-working domestic is kept up until the younger player returns home, the key not being allowed, or because now and then the game is not finished at one or two in the morning, and it thereby trespasses on the night's rest of him who has to be at his office by nine the following morning, why one had as well be isolated at once, and lead a Robinson Crusoe life. Where no further mischief is done than would be inferred by the supposed view of the case, it would be uncalled for to comment at all upon it. But in some cities billiards and card-playing are kept up all night, night after night, and till four and five o'clock in the morning. It may not be the mere sitting-up; it may not be the exchange of winnings and losings only; but it is the excitement, the great wear and tear of mind; why, there is more anxiety endured over a rubber, especially when bad with good play is united, or when fortune runs all on one side —or in a match at billiards—the stakes not making, perhaps, twenty shillings' difference during the night—or even at backgammon, chess, or any other game, than there is absolutely in a day's competition in the business of life, where hundreds change hands. Nero fiddled when Rome was burning; kings have been checkmated on the board and their throne at the same moment; and such is the fascination of cards and dice, that fortunes are often risked on a "turn-up." Once allow this sort of excitement to get the mastery, and health begins to ooze out at your fingers' ends.

Essays have been written on gambling, and all have denounced its withering influence. "Yes," exclaims B, "but you don't call a rubber, or a game at vingt-un, or any other round game, at which, besides, ladies play, gambling?" The man who is so phlegmatic as to be indifferent to, or disinclined to take a hand at, cards, should refuse every invitation he receives. He is only asked on the condition of making himself generally agreeable or useful. I have no fault to find with the player who, to oblige the host, parts with a score of shillings, by filling an opposite corner to an indifferent or inattentive player—that alone is vexing enough; but I certainly object to six hours at short whist, or making one at a round game where, stimulated by as many hours' drinking and smoking, that, with one and the other, the eye can scarcely travel across the table, and the mind is wrought up to a degree of irritability that bitterly bespeaks the sacrifice for the amusement. Morbid excitement, or excitement to excess of any kind, and that especially indulged in by young men—no matter whether card-playing, pool, sing-song, boating, spreeing, or larking, or whatever else carries the mind beyond the soberness of propriety, is most hurtful, and such of my readers as have faith in my counsel, and who prefer placid feelings, mental contentment, and good health, or who are seeking to gain these desiderata, I say unto them—AVOID ALL KINDS OF MORBID EXCITEMENT.

CHAPTER V.

SUMMARY.

HAVING gone through, in a purposely conversational, and, I hope, intelligible manner, the very important considerations of eating and drinking, and having made my passing remarks upon the various substances and fluids which form our dietary, I will beg a little farther attention to a kind of summary or recapitulation of how I would advise invalid and delicate persons to live; what I would have them to be careful of, and what I think they should avoid; how much, in a general way, they should take; and when, and how frequently, they should put it in practice. I will then conclude this part of my subject by the presentation of a few tables, adapted to the several degrees of INVALIDISM.

The natural and uppermost question a patient puts to his medical man, after having received his instructions about medicine, is, " Well, doctor, how am I to live?" The reply is usually, " Oh! sparingly—temperately; be careful. You must avoid spirits—take your medicine—and let me see you again." " May I eat meat?"

"Y e-e-s, only moderately." "May I take exercise?" "Ye-e-s, yes." "May I—I had something else to say, but I have forgotten it. Good day." And thus ends the colloquy; and how little wiser is the patient for his instructions. The medicine may be admirably prescribed, and excellently adapted for the case.

If there be any virtue in physicking by measure, there surely must be in dieting by the same principle. A pill, or draught, or powder, or dose of some sort or other, is advised to be taken every three, four, or six hours; and should not food and drink be taken with similar regularity? The only interpretation I can put upon the seeming fact is that, it would appear, if a man fall ill, he has only to take some nauseous stuff, and he will or will not, as it may turn out, get well. The study of diet is left to the public to learn, as they would astronomy and chymistry, if they would desire to be more learned than their neighbors. We are all fashioned so differently, that there are extremes of every kind; some people can digest anything, while others are compelled to hesitate before they take a mouthful. The multitude, however, are influenced by common laws. In a general way, certain articles of diet are generally indigestible, and over-feeding produces corresponding results to the strong and the weak, in proportion to the excess. These facts are ascertained only by experience. Youth lifts us over many difficulties. The appetite is the only guide, and the stamina of a growing boy helps him over the abuse which an elder person dare not commit. Many youthful habits are continued some time with impunity, that would be followed by serious inconveniences ten years afterward. It is very common to observe young persons drink off a tumbler of water or beer before commencing their dinner, which, although it may gratify a little morbid thirst, necessarily interferes with the digestion of the forthcoming meal; it distends the stomach, dilutes the gastric juice, and is a shock to the nervous tone of the stomach. Many elder persons commit the same error; but it is difficult to persuade them that it is an error, and that the flatulence and weight after the subsequent meal is the result of the water or drink taken beforehand. Abernethy forbade his patients to drink at all at dinner-time; and it will presently be seen that drink, at that period, is not only unnecessary, but also, as has been shown above, very prejudicial, and, if obstinately persisted in, ultimately productive of disease.

Consequently, as I observed before, unless there be specific instructions how to live given with the physic that is ordered to be taken, the treatment is sadly imperfect; and it is too much to expect the patient to know by inspiration how he should diet himself to get well, when probably it was only his careless living, of which he was ignorantly guilty, that caused his illness. Even the reform from intemperate habits, the relinquishment of spirituous drinks—in a word, teetotalism, unquestionably the greatest step ever made in a nation toward the improvement of health and security of universal happiness—how was it achieved (say to the wonderful extent it has already been)? Not by the preaching of the parsons, or by the advice and writings of the doctors, whose almost exclusive province it was, but by philanthropic individuals, by men chiefly from the humbler classes, who made the discovery themselves, and became the leaders of others. If any man, living or dead, deserves the benedictions of his fellow-creatures, Father Mathew is that man. It was not his position as a priest which gave him power; it was his homely, his common-sense, understandable exposition of the injurious consequences of drink, to both the mind and body, to the home, to the family, and to the self of the drunkard, that enabled him to lead the thousands to the shrine he himself worshipped, namely, Temperance. But while giving him credit for the change that he has effected, for the moral triumph he has gained, and the misery he has averted, his scheme is not wholly unattended with certain inconsistencies. Father Mathew, I presume, is not a physiologist, nor is teetotalism founded upon physiological principles; else wine, spirits, and beer, would not be entirely excluded from the table of man. Teetotallers admit that they may be taken medicinally; but medicine is usually administered to persons only when ill. Now, stimulatives are allowedly useful, not only in illness, but to prevent illness. There are some individuals who can not subsist without stimulatives; they are not unwell, but they would be liable to become so, if denied, *in toto*, the prohibited *stimuli*. It is difficult, I admit, to keep people within bounds; and perhaps the best way to avoid mischief on a large scale is to disallow spirits, &c., altogether, merely permitting the exceptions to infringe the rule. But of this as we go on; the advantages as well as disadvantages should be equally exhibited, and then those who infringe the laws of nature as well as of man, knowing beforehand the punishment in store, have only themselves to thank for their pains, and they deserve no commiseration.

"How am I to live?" I will presume the preceding leaves have been read; that the reader recollects what he has perused; that he carries away with him a general idea of what has been said about solids and fluids; that he remembers I disclaim against gross and careless feeding; that drinking and dissipation undermine and destroy the strongest constitution: that the picture of early improvidences has not been presented in vain; and that, at once and for all time, those errors which he has been addicted to he resolves to forego, to abandon, to forget; that the instructions as hitherto given, and presently to be offered, for better conduct, accord with his taste; and that the mere question of "How AM I TO LIVE?" is not put for idle curiosity, but to elicit an answer that shall, indeed, be a "Guide to health and long life," and which guide, if the responsibility of the case rests on my shoulders, i fthe patient be my patient, he will follow.

Burton, in his quaint and elaborate work "On Melancholy," considers the cure of disease to depend upon the six following conditions:—

  Diet,   Air,   Sleep,
  Retention, Exercise, Passions.

He suggests no mean addendum, which tells two ways—an obedient and liberal patient, and a skilful and honorable physician.

His notions are no diversion from the plan I have pursued in this book; but it is well to show what has herein been offered is supported by so good an authority.

Summary of Diet and Regimen, with Remarks.

In summer, rise at six or earlier; in winter, not later than seven. If your pursuit confine you within doors all day, take an hour's exercise the first thing in the morning. If it prove wearisome to walk before breakfast, provide yourself with a biscuit or crust, or if you can get it and need it, a cup of coffee. If you reside in the country, pursue the same plan. A light breakfast afterward will refresh you, and remove all fatigue. If you once commence the habit, you will find it more difficult to leave off than you found it to begin. A cold shower-bath, health permitting it, in the morning, is most salutary. It is no use, however, in taking it only occasionally; it should be used daily, in all weathers, and all the year round. Where that is not practicable, cold ablution, or sponging the body and chest, particularly, with cold water, or deluging the head in a "bucket from the well," is sure to do good. These are such agreeable processes, that one day's omission will occasion such a want of comfort, that the habit of persistence will become a delight to you.

I have offered a few comments on the beauties of bathing, generally, elsewhere, but no person should pass his or her life, without taking, for purposes of cleanliness and health, where it be practicable, a *warm bath* at least once a fortnight—certainly once a month; but it would not be unwise nor dangerous, as by many it is foolishly feared, once a week—but read the chapter presently.

If the weather be unfavorable, and you cannot go out, there are various means of taking exercise within doors: pacing a passage or room, with windows open; some light game, skipping, battledore, and shuttlecock. dumb-bells, fencing. A man in search of health must not mind being laughed at for seeming puerility. Even singing or reading aloud, or the practice of declamation, are severally serviceable. The most salutary of all early movements is a ride on horseback. A city business man may easily ride ten miles before breakfast. The immense benefits of sleeping out of town I have already expatiated upon; and the morning ride in the fresh air furnishes you with health and strength that will carry you through the day. We now come to the eating part.

Breakfast is usually the first meal. Some people, from habit—from suppers, perhaps—although early-risers, do not breakfast until eleven o'clock, when they will have a chop and a mug of ale. It is impossible to furnish such rules as shall be universally applicable. Dr. Combe ridicules the idea of fixed dietaries, or, indeed, prohibitions or allowances of any kind, inasmuch as men differ so in their capacities and appetites, that scarcely two individuals will be found whom the same regimen will suit. And where, therefore, man is master of himself, and his means can command anything he requires out of the common routine, he can the better study his feelings, which he is perfectly justified in doing.

However, this principle is good, that as we require both solids and fluids, it is better to adapt our resources to our wants; the first meal required is necessarily a fluid one, from the exhaustion we sustain during the night by perspiration, and the escape of other secretions. Like the earth, we need moisture; and instinct dictates that the commencement and close of the day are the best periods for partaking of it, and that those times render the enjoyment most congenial to our feelings, and productive to our personal comfort.

The materials of the tea-table are very simple in this country but epicures convert it into a déjeuné à la fourchette. The ordinary breakfast consists of tea or coffee, with bread and butter, or toast, to which is occasionally added eggs, fried ham or bacon, cold meat, chickens, &c.; but usually the appendages are taken but sparingly of; indeed, except one has to wait till a five o'clock dinner, or to undergo much exercise or fatigue, the quieter the breakfast the better. A very hearty breakfast is difficult to dispose of; it is productive, especially if three or four cups of liquid be swallowed, of much flatulence and eructations, with a degree of puffiness that continues disagreeable for the next two or three hours. Exercise should not be taken immediately after a good breakfast. It is advisable also to drink slowly, as well as to eat slowly. The stomach becomes more reconciled to a fluid meal when introduced gradually, than when poured in all of a heap; the thirst is better allayed, and the palate better satisfied. In selecting what we should drink for breakfast, we must be governed by our individual experience. Many people cannot take either tea or coffee, in which case, cocoa, or chocolate, or broma, or milk and water, or boiled milk with bread, or farinaceous food, or oatmeal porridge, or whatever else the ingenuity of the housewife or nurse may suggest, or the palate of the individual may fancy. From half to three quarters of a pint is sufficient, with a round or round and a half of toast, buttered when cold, the allowance to be increased according to appetite and circumstance ; a reasonable time for breakfasting is between eight and nine.

The next function of life which is most universally exercised immediately after breakfast, is the evacuation of the bowels. This affair is one of very great importance, and which no morbid delicacy should suffer to be disregarded. It is an ordination of nature, and a sure sign of something wrong when not obeyed. Constipation is a very marked symptom of indigestion, and may be looked upon as an indication that the diet is of too dry a nature, too astringent, or that the bowels are irritable, that the stomachic and intestinal secretions are at fault. So formidable an interruption to health, and so productive is constipation of general uneasiness, that various methods, dietetical, medical, and mechanical, are from time to time suggested for its relief; but the very remedies only keep up the disease, and, when once resorted to, cannot be dispensed with. Many people never obtain an evacuation of the bowels without medicine, or the use of the lavement, whereas the only two certainties to procure efficient relief are watchful living and exercise, both of which are miserably neglected. When possible, an evacuation should be secured ; the daily habit of visiting the closet at the same hour is a method very likely to insure success, and the practice cannot be too much insisted upon with regularity in early life ; among the dietetic provocatives, apart from simplicity of feeding, is the brown bread instead of white, and the unfermented (where it can be obtained or made) in preference to that prepared with yest.

Constipation is indeed a great nuisance, but it is always confirmed by medicine-taking rather than cured by it. When once the bowels become regular, be wise, and never take another purgative pill or dose but upon stern necessity. Constipation is mere irritation, inducing deficient secretion, and morbid apathy or positive constriction of the rectum and bowels generally.

The next consideration is how the time between breakfast and dinner should be filled up. If my publication be read by the man of business, he can better answer the question than I can; if by one, happily, controller of his own time, and one in search of health, I need scarcely say, that from ten till two is the best and most agreeable time for taking pedestrian or equestrian exercise. The ride by steamboat, railroad, or omnibus, or even foot journey, to the city or house of business, is of incalculable advantage, but how much more so is the liberty the uncontrolled man possesses of rambling out either in the green fields, on the cheerful river, or in the highways and byways of this beautiful world. From two to three hours thus spent daily, makes our stay here an elysium. It furnishes the meal for the soul, if I may be allowed such an expression, and which I employ without prejudice; the mind is gladdened—the perception brightened—and contentment reigns throughout. It completes the process of the transmutation of the food we consume into the blood that animates the mortal man—it is the last handiwork of nature in digestion. How blest, indeed, is he, and also ought he to feel, who possesses the inestimable privilege of having all things made to his desires—of being born to live, not to struggle—and of serving others rather than needing service himself. This is not the language of discontent, it is from one who believes *whatever is, is right;* and one who, from the naturally restricted privileges of a working bee, the more duly appreciates the freedom of a day's holiday—the ramble abroad, where the only buffets he encounters are those of the friendly breeze, and the only homage he is called upon to pay, the cheerful thanksgiving to the only Master he serves.

Exercise, in whatever shape availed of, in the bustle of trade, or the sports of the field, or in any of the other duties or pleasures of life, is indispensable to secure health.

The question of "Have you been out to-day?" presupposes generally that the morning was the time selected; it certainly has its advantages; but where it cannot be obtained in the forenoon, the remaining half of the day is amply sufficient to make man content. The afternoon jaunt and the evening stroll have severally admirers, and it is well we can not all select the same time, else we should jostle each other. The weather and seasons forbid and invite alternately, and circumstances must guide us in our selection.*

---

* Bathing is a great preservative to health, and as such deserves a separate article. The reader will find it further on.

SUMMARY.

The dinner should be the substantial, the nourishing meal of the day. One strong reason why it should be taken early in the day, in preference to late in the evening, is, that as the food has to be digested as well as swallowed, and which former requires some energy for its purpose, the meal ought to be taken before man is exhausted by the fatigues of the day, besides to allow time for the necessary exercise which should accompany the completing process of digestion.

The stomach, in shape, corresponds with the outline, which represents a section. In structure it resembles a pig's or sheep's bladder, except that it is rather thicker, from its more evident muscularity. It is capable of containing *three or four pints* of fluid or substances; it is made up of several coats, to each of which

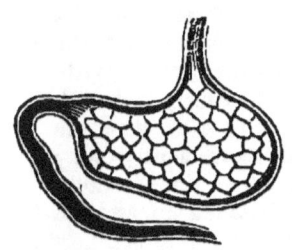

a name is assigned. The stomach has two openings, one for the reception of food, and the other for its exit, when sufficiently digested. The diagram below shows the place of the stomach in the abdomen, and the relative position of the other principle viscera.

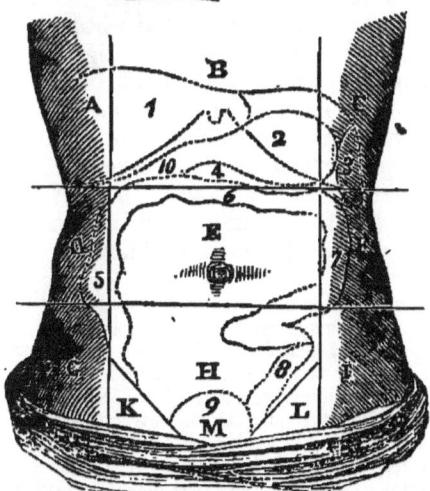

A. and C. The Hypochondriac Region.
B. E. Epigastric.
D. and F. Iliac.
E. Umbilical.
G. and L The Lumbar.
H. Hypogastric.
K. and L. The Ingual.
M. The Vesical.
1. The Liver.
2. Stomach.
3. Spleen.
4. Pancreas.
5, 6, and 7. The course of the large intestine, called the Colon.
8. The Rectum.
9. The Bladder.
10. The opening of the stomach in the small intestines, which occupy the central part of the abdomen.

Digestion usually takes from four to five hours before it is completed; the time is not invariably the same with everybody. With some the process is much more rapid; with others double the time is occupied. The stomach all this time is absolutely at work. Happily, except in disease, we are ignorant of what is going forward, scarcely cognizant we have a stomach; and there is certainly in health no feeling to tell us exactly whereabout it is situated.

It is, however, as well to know so much of anatomy, that if we should experience a twinge we might form some idea which part of our digestive machinery was attacked. I have hitherto presumed it to be of less importance that a reader should be rendered anatomically learned, than that he know simply what the office of the stomach was, and also have some idea of its powers. The annexed sketches, however, will convey at a glance a very good idea of the shape and relative position of the different organs concerned in the internal economy of man, and thereby rectify any omission.

Now it follows, and the policy is borne out in the universal maxim, that it is better to finish one thing first before we commence another, and so it is with digestion. Digestion is a specific process that involves certain duties, that cannot well be performed if subject to interruptions or additional imposts. The stomach, on receipt of the food, supplies promptly, that is to say, it secretes or pours forth from its surface a certain and limited amount of a powerful solvent fluid, called gastric juice; this mingles with the food, and rapidly dissolves the portion it comes in contact with. To render the contact more general, the stomach is furnished with a power of contracting upon itself, and squeezing, as it were, the food from one part to another. When the food is sufficiently pulpy or dissolved, it passes onward to the intestines, where the nutritious portion which is to form the blood of the body is taken up, and the extraneous carried forward and given off in the usual manner.*

Now it is well known that every act and movement of the body, or even exercise of the senses, is followed more or less with fatigue, and there is no reason why the stomach should not have a little breathing time, after having completed its work, as well as the legs and arms. Such a respite is necessary; and hence the prudence of allowing a little time to elapse beyond when the digestion is supposed to be completed, before fresh work is imposed. A quiet breakfast, being a fluid meal, is disposed of in perhaps three hours; therefore, if taken at eight or nine o'clock, dinner may follow at

---

* A writer on hydropathy, Dr. Johnson, disputes this theory, and contends that, in health, the food is wholly taken up in the system, and that the fœcal evacuations are entirely ordinary secretions, and that it is only where digestion is imperfect that the food passes through undissolved. This is very plausible, for in healthy evacuations there is no distinguishing what the diet has consisted of, whether fish, fowl, or meat, the color alone determining whether it was solid or fluid—milk or malt; whereas, in ill-health and faulty digestion, meaty fibres, certain vegetables and fruits, pass away scarcely altered. There is no doubt that the better the health, the more perfect the intermixture of the food in the system at large, and the evacuations consequently bespeak the tone of the powers of assimilation.

one or two. If protracted beyond that time, to five or six ; or later, some little refreshment is advisable, proportioned, of course, to the exercise and bustle going on. Lunches, else, are tantalizing interruptions, and except necessary to prevent faintness or exhaustion, had better be dispensed with. Besides, the materials of the lunch are usually some sweet or spongy substance—a bun, tartlet, or biscuit, with a glass of wine. It must be told that there is as much ceremony in digesting a mouthful as in a meal; and the digestive process being set in motion too quickly, enervates its powers, and disturbs the sympathies of appetite and relish that are usually in attendance when in a healthy condition.

Frequently and little, or much and seldom, must be adopted according to each man's capacity, of which, as I have observed before, every person should judge for himself. It is so easy to find out which best agrees ; but if the order be reversed, overfeeding or underfeeding are the consequences; there is less fear from the latter than the former. Now, with regard to the dinner, *it should be eaten slowly, and masticated thoroughly*, and the grand rule regulating the whole should be, *that we do not eat too much*. It has been said, we should only eat when we are hungry :—

> " When hunger calls, obey, nor often wait
> Till hunger sharpen to corrosive pain."

Exactly so ; but regularity in the dinner hour allows time for the gathering of the appetite, and also prevents the sufferings of delay.

An English dinner is usually made up of fish and meat, with vegetables, preceded or followed by pies or puddings, and accompanied with bread, wine or beer, with condiments. In health, nothing better than this fare can be found, supposing no excess of any one thing mentioned be committed ; and it is, therefore, left for all rational persons to partake of; and when indulged in with moderation only, there is little fear of the grace of

> " May good digestion wait on appetite,"

not being realized. Persons in feeble health must vary their table fare according to the instructions already given, or they may select it from the diet tables which will be found at the end of this article. The propriety of drinks at dinner is a matter of opinion. Unquestionably, dinner being a solid meal, requires only so much fluid as shall help to relieve the *dryness* of the repast, or to aid its miscibility ; but then there is almost sufficient moisture in the meat and vegetables for that purpose, and in the salivary and other secretions. If the said dryness prevail, and man's aptitude requires it, there is no reason why drink should altogether be excluded; and I should say, there can be no great harm in half a pint of mild table ale, or even stout or beer, if experience bespeak the necessity. When the digestion is feeble, and persons seem to need it, from one to three glasses of wine may be taken if preferred. These dietetic instructions to one in health may well be laughed at; to the sick man, the case is different; and as to him they are chiefly addressed, allowances must be made for this wearisome minuteness. With regard to taking stimulants in the shape of wine and beer at dinner, or at any time, by the healthy or by the sick, a main consideration is, do they *excite?* or, on the other hand, do they *produce lethargic feelings?* The mere exhilaration of spirits, the cheerfulness which follows, or the general comfortable sensations which prevail after wine, beer, or spirits, do not determine that mischief is going on, nor should a man be always feeling his pulse to know whether his life is running too fast; but there are other indications which cannot be mistaken—the sensible increased beating of the heart, the throbbing in the forehead, the evidence of powerful mental excitement, the flurry following a quickened step, the confusion of thought, the puffiness and general distension—all of these, and many more, known by experience to the free liver, determine the mischievous tendency of stimulants, and prove, by the absence of these feelings, when not partaken of, that they had better be avoided.

Dining is a much more important affair than many people suppose. It is true a hungry stomach is a most unruly fellow, and a man is up in arms if compelled to go without his dinner; but it is often looked upon as the mere link between body and life, and it is considered sufficient so long as we can fill our stomachs. Now, there are certain conditions, if we desire really to benefit by the meal, that should be observed, independently of regularity and a wholesome supply of the daily fare. Nothing is so injurious as hurried eating, or proceeding to dine when overheated or fatigued. There are many persons in cities, who allow themselves not more than half an hour to *run* to their dinner, consume it, and *run* back again. Many there are also, who defer it till hunger pinches their bellies; and on the strength of a good appetite exhaust themselves by a five or six miles ride, or corresponding walk home to join the dinner table, and by the time the repast is over, they are absolutely fitter to go to bed than remain up for several hours, in which lethargy the stomach joins, and digestion is more or less suspended. I have elsewhere observed on the necessity of dinner being a cheerful meal, and also of its not being taken immediately after exertion;

at least a quarter of an hour's respite is advisable. It is equally imprudent to return to active duty without a corresponding pause after, as well as before.

Supposing little drink be taken at dinner. and allowing from three to four hours for its digestion, a fluid meal comes in very *apropos* at this time ; and by its miscibility, completes the solution of the food, and facilitates its transmission into the bowels. Tea, therefore, may be taken about this time. The comfortable and refreshing feelings which ensue test the propriety of the repast.*

As we are not merely sent here to feed and repose, but to fulfill various other duties, among which recreation as well as toil has its demands, custom has assigned the evening for general pastime and association among each other ; and, accordingly, the body being hereby invigorated, the mind is fitter for its lighter occupation. The pursuits of the evening are multifarious ; to dictate which amusement should be followed would be trespassing upon other people's tastes, which is beyond the privilege of a writer on dietetics ; certain it is, that exercise should form a part. The walk out and home and family dance are alike serviceable ; and where the one be impracticable, the other should not be dispensed with.

An early dinner admits of a light supper, but it should be taken by weight and measure. The tempting things put upon table often induce one to eat more than is wholesome ; and it is indeed a wretched recompense for the short-lived gratification of pleasing the palate by an extra plate or a glassful, of having to pass a night of nightmare and hideous dreams ; besides, the punishment is extended over the next day, by the feelings of lassitude consequent upon loss of rest.

I need not say a word about the unwholesomeness of hot meat suppers to a person in uncertain health : they are proverbially mischievous, and a man of any experience is rarely found to be a guest thereat. Of late hours I have already spoken at length. With regard to sleep, it should be remembered that ventilation of a sleeping apartment is of as much importance as that of the day-room, and hence it is well to choose large and lofty bed-rooms ; if the sleeper be not very susceptible of taking cold, I would advise the windows—or at least one of them, if there be more—to be kept half down during the night. Slumber should be sought for

---

* As general rules, tea had better be omitted where wine has been freely partaken of at dinner, and tea taken with or close upon dinner is alike an unfavorable mixture.

not later than ten or eleven o'clock by the valetudinarian, and he thereby may secure from eight to nine hours' rest, which are sufficient, and not too much, for the invalid, or for the preservation of health.

A happy and even temper, is an invulnerable shield against the misfortunes—worldly, bodily, and mental—of human life; and as I am convinced it can be acquired where not already possessed, it is a study I would urge every one in need of to carry out to the letter.

Thus may the twenty-four hours be passed; remembering, meantime, the hints furnished regarding the control of the passions, that no matter whatever the exercise of the mind or body may be, nature has its limits, and the transgression invariably draws down its punishment. The last words of Dr. Spurzheim were, that "man never will be happy till he learns God's laws, and has wisdom to obey them." If this aphorism be fairly carried out, and the trouble be taken to make the same our especial study, we shall assuredly escape the prickly thorns of a corrupt body or a distempered mind; and may at last—

> "Like ripe fruit drop
> Into our mother's lap, or be with ease
> Gathered, not harshly plucked."—MILTON.

CHAPTER VI.

DIETETIC RULES.

Low Diet.

Breakfast and " Tea."—Warm new milk and water—weak black tea, its astringent properties corrected by a due addition of milk. Gruel made with oatmeal, toast, or brown, household, or the unfermented bread, at least one day old, and without butter. Rusks sopped in the above fluids. The quantity of fluids of these meals should not exceed from half to three quarters of a pint. Of solids, from two to three ounces are sufficient.

Dinner.—Gruel, new milk and arrow-root, sago, or tapioca; chicken and veal broths, not exceeding half a pint; roast apples, light bread or rice puddings, not exceeding in bulk four ounces. Pastry of every description must be avoided.*

Supper.— Gruel, arrow-root; farinaceous food, four to six ounces.

Occasional Drinks. — Filtered or spring-water, toast-water, made with toasted bread or browned biscuit, barley-water, whey, lemonade of subdued acidity; sweet oranges may be freely taken if the sense of thirst be oppressive. Great regularity must be observed in taking these meals.

It is only in cases of extreme ill-health that this diet is advised.

Middle Diet.

Breakfast and " Tea."—Same as in "low diet," with the addition of mixed tea. Dry toast, made with brown† bread, where constipation prevails, or rusks, " captains' " biscuits.

---

* By *pastry* I mean custards, trifles, tartlets, sponge-cakes, puffs, buns, cheese-cakes. and similar abominations; the same interdiction applies equally to all other stages in a course of dieteties.

† *Brown Bread.*—Although it may be procured at every baker's, still there is a vast difference in its quality. Some bakers study to make it even more palatable than white bread, and endeavor to give it a biscuity flavor. To be genuine and effective for the end it is taken, it should be made as follows:

Take of wheat, ground, with all the bran left in it (to be had of the dealers),

Luncheon (if required).—A cup of isinglass, arrow-root, sago, tapioca, with a biscuit, or two or three bars of toasted (stale) bread.

Dinner.—In addition to " low diet," boiled chickens, calves' and sheep's feet stewed, mutton, chicken, and other broths, beef-tea, boiled soles, whiting, turbot, &c.; lamb, potatoes, asparagus, light bread, macaroni or rice pudding, roast apples. After the repast may be taken one glass of port, sherry, or Madeira wine, diluted with at least twice its quantity of water.

Supper.—A cup of gruel, sago, tapioca, or arrow-root. The same quantities should be observed in middle and full diet as in low diet—it is the quality which makes the difference.

Remarks.

Breakfast.—As a general rule, the solids, such as bread and butter, toast, biscuits, or what-not for breakfast, should not exceed from four to six ounces, nor should the liquids amount to more than from half to three-quarters of a pint, and the sense of comfort afterward must justify even so much. At tea-time the solids are scarcely requisite—one or two thin slices of bread and butter, or a couple of squares of cold buttered toast, are sufficient.

At *dinner*, half a pound to three quarters of substantials is usually sufficient, with perhaps six to eight ounces of water or mild beer; but drinks at dinner had better be avoided.

At *supper*, not exceeding from four to six ounces should be taken.

Now, it can not be too often stated, that the amount of strength to be acquired does not depend upon the quantity of food consumed, but entirely upon what only is digested, and nothing is more erroneous than to press a person to eat when there is no appetite. Nature takes away the appetite, because food, under the circumstances, would be highly dangerous; and the appetite only returns when the cause of the disease, the irritability from the disordered secretions, or even the specific inflammation that is present in illness, be

a peck; add half a pint of new yeast, as free from bitter as possible; mix with water rather warmer than new milk, making it like a thick batter in the middle of the pan; then allow it to rise; then mix a tablespoonful of salt with lukewarm water, and add to bulk, kneading all together; afterward allow it to stand about an hour; then divide it and place it in tins; lastly, put the loaves into a quick oven, where they will be done in about an hour and a half. This formula is given, although the unfermented bread is fast superseding it; but still, prejudices are not to be beaten out of us, and many persons cling to old customs, and have faith in yeast over soda and muriatic acid.

removed. It is true, the stomach may temporarily lose its tone, and require medical aid, such as tonics, to assist it, but they should be cautiously administered. The patient prays his physician to give him something to restore the appetite, and he will then soon be well, but the circumstances should be carefully looked into, before the request be complied with, and an artificial provocative be resorted to. Many a convalescent patient has been thrown back by the imprudent and premature exhibition of food and stimuli. "Middle diet" is best fitted for delicate persons, and such as have become ill from over-feeding, or run out of health from excesses of one kind or another.

Before giving directions what should regulate or constitute "full diet," I will offer a table which I will call "special diet," not so much for indiscriminate adoption of as for reference to those patients whom I may have occasion to advise in the course of my practice.

Special diet, for a nervously-debilitated Invalid.

Breakfast.—A teacupful of milk, say at seven o'clock, or a cup of porridge.* An hour's walk. At nine, one or two teacupfuls of black tea, with a round of brown bread, fermented or unfermented (one day old), toasted, and buttered when cold. If the walk can not be taken between the interval, the food and tea may be taken consecutively about eight or half-past, and exercise of some kind availed of a couple of hours afterward. If the weather forbid an out-door stroll, or the occupation prohibit relaxation of any kind, the next best substitute is walking up and down the room, and timing your perambulations, getting at least an hour between each meal, which would yield, possibly, during the day, a distance of half a dozen miles.

Dinner had better be taken about one or two o'clock; but where it can not be had until five or six, a lunch of a dry biscuit may be availed of, nor is there any great objection to a glass of sherry wine; but if the invalid find that it does not comfort, exhilarate, strengthen, or otherwise benefit, or other reasons exist why it should

---

* Scotch porridge forms an excellent repast. The true Scotch oatmeal should be obtained, and the best way of mixing it is as follows: Take about four tablespoonfuls of the oatmeal and add the same quantity of water or milk; mix them well together; then add half a pint of cold water or milk; and boil the same, stirring it during the time; boil for two minutes, or until it thickens, and add salt or sugar to please the palate. This will be found an excellent breakfast and tea, or supper, and will keep the bowels in healthy action.

not be taken, an entire abstinence from that or any other fluid will not harm.

The dinner may consist of two fair slices of warm fresh meat, with one or two potatoes, or where much flatulence prevails, without vegetables of any kind, for a time, but a round of brown bread; this may be followed by a small supply of any light pudding, such as baked rice, plain bread, macaroni, or other similar puddings. Where the digestion is feeble, meat may be taken only on alternate days, and poultry or fish, if it agree, the other days. In cases of chronic debility I have found not over-dressed curries a great help —a chop curried—part of a fowl—rabbit—piece of veal, or any light digestible substance served up in that form; it stimulates wholesomely the stomach, and forms an occasional good substitute for, or addendum to, the family joint. The rice served up with it softens the pungency of the curry powder, but potatoes may be used instead, if preferred. An invalid epicure may find the subjoined recipe serviceable to advise his cook thereon. Bread should be freely eaten, where vegetables are disallowed. Except thirst prevail, drink of all kinds had better be avoided; but, if justified by experience, one or two glasses of sherry may be taken. No fixed rule can be laid down concerning drink at dinner; but on an average, the meal is digested better without a drop, there being plenty in the viands constituting the dinner.

Tea may be taken about three or four hours after dinner—and may consist of two or even three cupfuls of black tea, provided no drink be taken at dinner, and that it be not found to disagree, otherwise tea is apt to check digestion rather than assist it, producing flatulence, sleeplessness at night, and many nervous feelings. When an invalid dines at five o'clock, very many stomachs can not dispense with an after solid repast; experience, however, must decide the point whether such be required. A biscuit, slice or two of toast, or a cup of gruel, are the best substitutes for substantials. No smoking, snuffing, " grogging," or wine-bibbing, allowed; and the excuse for the occasional infringement, namely, that of an old friend dropping in, is an untenable one.

Now come we to " full diet," which is to be allowed to persons requiring strength, and blessed with natural, good, and increasing appetites.

Full Diet.

Breakfast and " Tea."—Same as in " middle diet;" in addition to which may be taken coffee or chocolate; toast or stale bread, but very sparingly buttered.

Luncheon.—A biscuit and a glass of table ale or porter.

Dinner.—The "Middle Diet" bill of fare may be augmented by boiled lamb, chickens, mutton chop, rump-steaks, roast or boiled fresh meats, curries, light bread puddings, the fruit of pies (avoiding the pastry) baked or boiled rice or tapioca puddings. At this meal, table beer, *pale ale*, or porter, may be taken as common drink; sherry or a couple of glasses of port, or Madeira, carefully noting the symptoms produced by their effect.

Supper.—Same as in "Middle Diet."

An additional glass of wine at dinner, or at luncheon, will convert this "full" into "generous" diet.

A very important desideratum to all dyspeptics, especially those adopting this diet, is a good set of teeth, particularly the "grinders," which, unfortunately, few individuals possess—the loss of which may be attributable to their complaint; it being observed, that persons with weak stomachs are seldom free from the anguish arising from decaying teeth. The contrivances of art now-a-days render the loss of natural teeth of minor importance; and I would strongly recommend the invalids, where necessary, to resort to them without delay. It is, however, very important to be particular whom to apply to.

The tartar on the teeth is nothing more than the chymical deposit of the saliva; hence the safety of cleansing the teeth and rinsing out the mouth after *every* meal. The teeth should be especially brushed *every night*, and well washed in the morning, to dislodge all collections of food.

Milk, Farinaceous, Vegetable, and Fruit Diet.

The articles of food within this range are milk, eggs lightly boiled, gruel, farinaceous food, sago, arrow-root, tapioca, isinglass, wheaten and barley bread, rice, potatoes, carrots, parsnips, turnips, peas, artichokes, cauliflowers, cabbage, spinach, water-cress, celery. Fruits and farinacea are recommended by some writers as the only necessary food for man, but the world recognizes man as an omnivorous animal, and hence fruits have, like meat and vegetables, their especial place. Stone-fruit, as nectarines, apricots, peaches, plums, and cherries, are the least digestible, and should never be taken but when ripe; apples and pears are not so apt to run into the acetous fermentation as stone fruit, but unless ripe and well masticated, had better be eaten cooked. Oranges, gooseberries (avoiding the skins), grapes without the husks and seeds, currants, ripe strawberries, and raspberries, follow consequently in the order in which they are enumerated, the first being most easy of digestion. Notwithstanding such an ample store of materials, the selection must of course depend upon season, appetite, and the known effects of each upon individual constitutions. The list is given to save the invalid the trouble of ferreting his memory of what enters into the composition of this diet, which is frequently recommended, and found particularly serviceable to weak and delicate stomachs.

Directions for making Curry.

Cut up a rabbit or fowl into small pieces, then slice two onions and three grains of garlic, add two dozen coriander-seed, and fry it in a quarter of a pound of fresh butter until brown; then add the rabbit or fowl, with two large tablespoonfuls of the curry powder, and a half a pint of water, and a little salt; stew it gently until the meat be tender; take it out, and add to the gravy two boiled mashed potatoes, and then pour it over the meat; afterward take a pound of curry-rice, and boil it slowly with a teaspoonful of salt, until the grain becomes soft, then border the dish with it.

N. B.—Be sure and strain the rice very dry.

CHAPTER VII.

LIEBIG'S THEORY ON LIFE, HEALTH, AND DISEASE.

"An important chapter."—AUTHOR.

"But why and wherefore, ask ye, such things are?
Nor is it wondrous ye should seek to know
As well what they should be, as why winds blow.
It would save much logic, if, with with female tact,
We stood upon a truth—a fact's a fact;
But, lest such independence should offend,
To my poor exposition pray attend."—OLD TALE.

How often does an invalid find himself bemoaning over his condition, wondering within his own mind what can be the matter with him! If he have a watch that stops, or gets out of order, he takes it to the maker, and is contented to learn that it wants cleaning, or that the spring is broken, and he leaves it with the artificer to effect the necessary reparation; but when ill himself, notwithstanding his doctor may tell him he has rheumatism, or indigestion, or that he is hypochondriacal, and that, like his watch, he wants cleansing and freshening up, and undertakes to do the same for him, still he is not so easily satisfied. If not righted within a few days, he gets impatient, and ponders over his malady—*What is rheumatism? whas is indigestion? and what is hypochondriacism?* If the recent invalid thinks in this manner, how much more does the conjecture worry the confirmed invalid—he who has been ailing for time—not weeks and months only, but years; he who is so feeble as to be scarcely able to stand—whose heart beats ready to burst on the slightest exertion and excitement—whose breath appears denied him—although in the prime of life! How natural is it that such a person should exclaim, "Woe is me!" and that he should like to know what really *is* the matter with him—what, in fact, his disease is, and why he should be singled out as the sufferer, when he sees younger and older comrades free from similar annoyances. The category may be extended still further, and in his wanderings and wonderings he at last seeks to know, *What is life?*

And why should he not?—the problem is not so unsolvable. It certainly is as well to have some reasons for the faith which is within us; and it surely is consolatory to ascertain, if we cannot find out what life really is, at least how it is to be preserved; if not what pain actually be, at least what produces it; and if the philosophy of death be inexplicable, let us push our inquiries, which can be resolved, as to what retards its approach.

The object of the preceding pages has been in a great measure to achieve all this, but it has relied upon facts—it has taught the value of this and that diet—it has urged the necessity of fresh air and exercise—it has dwelt upon the policy of avoiding excesses—all truisms in their way, but unfortunately hitherto taught only as lessons by rote.

The solutions to the inquiries of what is life and what is disease, may do more—they may teach principles; and if the explanation, which I am about to offer, be intelligible and correct, the truth and utility of the code presented, not only of *what to eat, drink, and avoid*, but how to live, that all may reach the top of "threescore and ten," will be strongly and easily impressed upon the least reflective mind.

It is one thing to know *what* tends to the maintenance and preservation of health, but another to know the why and wherefore; and it is presumed it will considerably strengthen the mind of the timid invalid or the skeptical valetudinarian, if it can be shown *why* gross, inappropriate, or insufficient feeding be injurious, and *wherefore* fresh air, exercise, and rest, should be such a curative for the ailments of mortality, and a preservative for the healthy man.

Addressing my work in homely phraseology for the homely purpose of advising such as may not be chymically learned in the different properties of food and drink, and also those who may not have made the study of their economy a feature to this time, it might almost appear that the present chapter, seemingly leaning to metaphysical theories, is superfluous, that I and my book are attempting to carry our readers out of their depth; but I will rely upon the combined sagacity of my friends and myself to avoid such a fatal immersion. I am not about to promulgate any novel doctrine of my own coinage, nor one that shall insist upon fallacies in past times, but it would exhibit great remissness in the author of such a publication as this professes to be, were he to withhold (which, if he did, might be construed into "that he did not know") from the public what is passing as recognized notions among his own professional contemporaries on this very important and inter-

LIEBIG'S THEORY ON LIFE, HEALTH, AND DISEASE.

esting subject—principles not only influencing how to avoid disease, but how to cure it. Shakspeare has familiarized us with the seven ages of man, from the cradled child to toothless decrepitude; but the tenure of life is held upon the same terms with the infant at the breast as the old man at seventy, namely, by feeding and breathing. The value of fresh air, careful living, and exercise, were appreciated in the days of the "bard for all time."

The same materials and combinations would have formed gas and steam a thousand years ago, that yield them now, and the principles of life have not altered since the creation, but it has fallen to the lot of modern times to give the new reading to their *modus operandi*, or economy in detal.

To Liebig, of Giessen, the leviathan in chymistry of the present century, are we mainly indebted for the prevailing theory:—

1st. It is, that the human body is determined in its configuration by a property inherent with its existence, denominated *vis vitæ*, or *vital force*, (or say *life itself*, if preferred), but of which, beyond the truth of its presence, we are ignorant.

2dly. That our existence is dependent upon chymical operations;

3dly. That the human body is its own laboratory, wherein it generated its own heat;

4thly. That it is constantly consuming and giving *off* its own elements; and

Lastly. That it derives a renewal of the same from the nourishment supplied to it, and the atmosphere by which it is surrounded.

This is all plain sailing; amounting, in reality, that we live by eating, drinking, and breathing, which everybody can understand. But the phenomena about to be named, exhibit much originality of thought, and when understood, are strikingly evident.

The living human body is reducible, like all other matter, to its elementary principles; and as it is always undergoing waste or decomposition, it would soon consume itself, or, vulgarly speaking, die of inanition or starvation, were it not for the supply from without.

Liebig therefore says, that as a living body cannot form its own elements, they can only be derived from the food which contains them. The known elementary substances in all nature number between fifty and sixty, nearly a fourth of which are discovered in the human body.

The principal elements inhabiting the corporeal substance of man, and of which we have chiefly to do with in these details, are

| Oxygen, | Carbon, |
| Hydrogen, | Nitrogen, |

Therefore all food not containing especially these four elements* in combination is innutritious; and as nitrogen holds the more prominent place in the animal economy, as contributing to the formation of every part of the human body, no food amalgamates with the blood that does not possess it; hence the distinction between food called

Nitrogenized, or Nutritious.	Non-Nitrogenized, or Innutritious.
and	

This class includes—
  Bread,
  Meat, and all
  Vegetables,
which latter contains, though in a less degree, in corresponding bulk of bread and meat, the elements of the organized body.

This class includes, to the wonderment, perhaps, of many persons, such, especially, who have imbibed the notion that we could not do without them, namely:—
  Fat,   Wine,
  Gum,   Beer,
  Sugar, Spirits.

* In talking of elements, and giving the names of oxygen, hydrogen, and carbon, it is presumed the reader is acquainted, without giving a description of what they really are, beyond that they are elements. It must be admitted, that to a reader not conversant with the literal meaning of the terms, the statement cannot be very clear; for who among such can perceive the drift of being told that he is made up of nitrogenized atoms, when his own limited conception extends not beyond the fact of his being made of flesh and blood? A man may be a very sensible one without being a scientific one; but it is useless to prate about subjects, the premises of which are not understood. For the benefit of my thus far unlearned, but no less amiable and worthy readers, I will endeavor to define the meaning of the term elements. The earth and all things within it, upon it, and surrounding it, of animated and inanimated nature, including the atmosphere it floats in, have been found by chymists to consist of a certain number of substances, just as all the words which compose a language are resolvable into a few letters. These substances appear not to be further divisible, and hence they are termed *elements of matter*, or *simple bodies*. The majority are found only in combination with each other. These elements are chiefly divisible into gases, earth, and metals.

Notwithstanding the apparent difficulty, at the moment, of conceiving the possibility of resolving, say, for example, a deal table, a house, a brick, an instrument of music, a hat, or any object which presents itself, much less articles that we eat and drink, into their elements, still, the difficulty will vanish to any one at all conversant with the science of chymistry. Thus, oxygen and hydrogen (gases) form water. Nitrogen and oxygen (gases) are nearly the sole ingredients in atmospheric air; whereas, in different proportions, yet combined, they produce virulent poisons, such as nitric and nitrous acids. The rust on an iron nail is oxyde of iron. All our medicinal and chymical preparations consist of acids and alkalies, which are formed of combinations of elements, or, the natural productions of leaves, barks, fruit, &c., have a like basis. To bring the illustration nearer home, human fat, upon analysis, is reducible to the elements of carbon and oxygen, in the proportion of 120 parts of the former to 10 of the latter; and in order to afford a still further idea, the following table is extracted from Liebig's work,—to show the relative pro-

Nitrogen, or *azote*, enters into every organic or living substance.

Fat and water contain no nitrogen, and yet they are component parts of the animal body; but they are not considered *organized* or *living substances*.

Nitrogen, therefore, is indispensable for the development, growth, nutrition, and renovation of all living parts; consequently, it is only nitrogenized food that is capable of forming blood, and of contributing to the organized structures. Liebig gives to such food the name of *elements* of nutrition.

Non-nitrogenized food does not enter into the composition of blood, or contribute to animal life, but it is essential to health, as furnishing *carbon* and *hydrogen*, the oxydation of which develops heat: in fact, without the continual supply of non-nitrogenized portions of the elements we are especially dealing with in human composition, that are found to exist in the ordinary butcher's meat and the corn that yields us our daily loaf. Thus we have in one hundred parts of

	Meat.	Wheat.	Rye.	Oats.
Of Carbon	51.82	46.1	46.2	50.7
" Hydrogen	7.51	5.8	5.6	6.4
" Oxygen	15.10	43.4	44.2	36.7
" Nitrogen	21.37	2.3	1.7	2.2
" Ashes	4.20	2.4	2.3	4.0
	100.00	100.0	100.0	100.0

Carbon is a substantial element, and generally signifies charcoal—(the diamond is the clearer and more perfect illustration.) The carbon of human food, separable during assimilation or digestion, is analogous to the charred residue of the burnt log. The human body is reducible to thirteen elements, nine more than those already named; which, to spare further reference, are herein enumerated:—

Phosphorus,   *Fluorine,   †Calcium,
Sulphur,   †Potassium,   ‡Iron,
*Chlorine,   †Sodium,   ‡Manganese,

Those marked thus * are gases; thus † earth; ‡ metals; while phosphorus and sulphur are substances, like carbon, of neither class. Other elements have been detected, but only incidentally, such as alum, copper, magnesia, gold, lead, arsenic, &c. These additional elements are found in the various parts of our mortal selves: the metals in the blood; the earth in the bones; and others in the nerves, brain, &c.—(See Liebig's "Animal Chymistry.")

From the tables just given, it will be seen how large a portion of our ordinary food consists of carbon and oxygen; which, although occupying space in our organization, yet are ostensibly in a constant state of fusion, according to the theory, and thereby diffusing warmth throughout the body. Their escape, as before detailed, is effected by the secretions, which are constantly travelling towards the surface through the skin and lungs, and which are given off, whether the fresh supply comes in or not; which, if not forthcoming, the body, as stated, actually burns to death.

food, there would not be a sufficiency of carbon to check the influence of the oxygen upon the other elements of the body, and consequently we should die as in starvation—be literally burnt to death. Liebig calls non-nitrogenized food—elements of respiration. This explanation may appear to justify the imbibition of wine, beer, and spirits—but they exert another influence—they are locally mischievous taken to excess, and produce disturbance of action, creating irritation that breaks up the equilibrium of vital force presently to be described, and which is, in fact, disease; besides, also, there are other sources of carbon less destructive and more abundant, at less consumption, than wine, beer, or spirits. It will be remembered that in the preceding pages they have been considered merely as *stimulative*, not *nutritive*. The vital force is the property that not only determines the division of the body into legs and arms, but resists powerfully all alterations which caprice or accident may provoke; for obesity and leanness (both forms of disease) do occur. Heads can be flattened, as is done in some wild countries, noses and ears can be lengthened, and feet can be obstructed in their development, as we see among the Chinese; but these changes are all at the cost of natural resistance. We cannot turn a man into a horse, although we may impose upon him the labor of one!

It is *vital force* which propels the blood in its circulatory round throughout the body, which distributes the various secretions through their various ramifications, which provokes the exchange of the old materials in the reparation of the body for the new, which, in fact, regulates every voluntary or involuntary movement; and this *vital force* furthermore is influenced (within its own sphere) by the same laws which regulate all nature, such as gravitation, attraction, and repulsion, from the falling of a stone to the stumble of that glorious fabric—man!

The *materials* of life are held together by chymical cohesion and resistance. The principal phenomenon is *combustion*, which operation is perpetually, more or less, going on, by the *carbon* of the food and the *oxygen* of the atmosphere.

Carbon is the essential constituent of every living or organized tissue, both vegetable and animal; and Liebig supposes than an adult man consumes nearly a pound daily. The same *carbon* is disposed of, after having been *burnt* in the body, in its contact with oxygen, and escapes in equal quantity, except that unconsumed, and which goes to form fat, by the excretions, and principally by the exhalation from the lungs in the *form* of carbonic acid gas.

Oxygen abounds in all nature—the air we breathe, the water we drink, and the food we consume, all contain it. No function of life, or operation in nature, could exist or be fulfilled without it; it is oxygen which rusts iron, which tarnishes quicksilver, and which oxydizes other metals. It is the combination of oxygen that kindles the fire in the grate that illuminates our rooms, that contributes to the warring of the elements. Earth, water, air, and fire, would lose their identity without it; these are familiar examples. We could not live independently of it, nor are we able to breathe any atmosphere divested of it.

The following is the theory of animal heat:—Wherever a union of oxygen and carbon takes place, in whatever part of the body it may be, combustion ensues, and heat is thereby evolved.

Hence the warmth of the body is kept up according to our consumption of carbon, and the amount of oxygen we inhale, or otherwise consume. In cold and clear weather, oxygen abounding in proportion to the rarefaction of the atmosphere, the greater is the combustion and consequent abstraction of the carbon; hence, also, the greater necessity for its supply, and consequently, the greater appetite we experience to induce us to furnish the bodily fuel. This explains why the Esquimaux are such great feeders; and it furthermore proves that food and exercise are better and more permanent generators of warmth than clothing.

The fact can be attested by the feelings after a meal in the coldest weather; a simple illustration of the office of exercise is by provoking the circulation of the blood through benumbed fingers, which immediately glow with warmth, on being excited. Oxygen accompanies the circulation throughout the body, but where it is not freely distributed, which it is not when the equilibrium of the vital force is disturbed, as in cold fingers, the combustion alluded to does not, or only very feebly, take place, because the distribution of the oxygen thereto is retarded, but the moment the circulation recovers itself, then the combustion goes on as usual, and warmth is restored.

The body, like any other substance, has a tendency to accommodate itself to the temperature of the surrounding medium. It becomes cool, or increases in warmth accordingly; and hence the necessity of adapting the diet to preserve a uniformity of temperature, such as is consistent with health.

Clothing is merely an equivalent for food. In proportion to artificial warmth, the less is our appetite.

Liebig adds, if we were to go naked, and were exposed, as in savage life, to extremes of cold and fatigue, we should be able to consume immense quantities of whale blubber and tallow candles by the pound, or drink almost *ad libitum* brandy and train oil without bad effects, because the carbon and hydrogen thereby consumed would only meet the demand of the absorbed oxygen.*

Thus does he explain the injury of over and depraved feeding. An Englishman arrives in a hot climate—loses his appetite, and stimulates his stomach by spices and other hot provocatives; he eats as usual, but he does not get rid of it; or a Londoner may commit the same folly of overloading his system at home; the quantity of carbon accumulates; in the one instance, the temperature of the atmosphere forbids exercise, or does not allow a sufficient amount of oxygen to keep the quantity of carbon in subjection; and in the other, the love of ease and corporeal indulgence constitute similar hindrances. Disease in both instances ensues.

In England, these errors from excess of carbon are more prevalent in summer. In winter, the excess of oxygen prevails, and hence diseases of the lungs: a strong reason why persons prone to consumption should be generously supported in the cold months.

Regularity of living should not comprise the same weight and quantity of food daily, whether the day be fine or dry, or cold and clear, or warm and foggy, or whether exercise be taken or not; because under these circumstances the amount of oxygen does not correspond with the supply of carbon, for, as it has been observed, the oxygen prevails in cold and clear weather, and more is consumed in exercise than indolence; and the oxygen would then be in excess, whereas in damp weather, with indolent habits, it would be insufficient.

It has been calculated that a man receives about two pounds of oxygen daily; the same amount is given off again, whether he receive food or not, in combination with a part of his body, and accordingly, if he take no food, each day he must diminish in weight until all the consumable materials are disposed of. The duration of life under these circumstances is modified by the quietude observed, the state of the atmosphere, and the presence of water. On water alone persons have lived twenty days.

In starvation, not only is the fat consumed, but every other part of the body which is soluble goes to supply the imperative demands of the oxygen, taken in through the lungs; the muscles shrink and lose their contractibility, the brain itself at last yields to the intruder, and undergoes the process of oxydation, and delirium, mania, and death, close the scene. Decay is the result of a similar union with oxygen.

* This is well explained in the theory of starvation.

In all chronic diseases, death is produced by the same cause—the chymical action of the atmosphere.

Man and all other animals are exposed at every period of their lives to the unceasing and destructive action of the atmosphere. With every breath he expires a part of his body, every moment of his life he produces carbonic acid, the carbon of which his food must replace, or *he dies!*

THE FOLLOWING IS THE SUMMARY AND INFERENCES OF THE LIEBIGIAN THEORY.

That man derives his support from food analogous in elementary principles to his own composition.

That he is continually undergoing wear and tear, or, in other words, wasting* away on the one hand, and supplying the consumption on the other, so that when in health and at maturity, no diminution or increase in his weight is observed.

So continuous is this change going on, that every movement is the result of an alteration of structure—not a finger is raised, a glance taken, a thought given birth to, without a change—without a wear and tear of the material wherein abides the function. In proportion to the intensity of the feeling or movement, so is the change in the organization. It then can easily be conceived how injurious must excess of any one manifestation of human life be, much more when many are combined, whether such be fatigue of body or abuse of mind. Hence the seeming fact of many men looking old at mid-life, and others, who have been careful, looking younger than they really are.

In stating that every word, thought, or deed, involves a consumption of material is only re-echoing what hitherto physiologists calculated upon taking place in cycles of three years, namely—an entire change in every particle of the human body—so that we retain at the expiration of that time not an atom of our former self. This is very probable when we reflect upon the constant, though necessary metamorphosis of structure or tissues we are subjected to in the scheme being detailed. It is the *vital force* that preserves our positive facial identity.

Liebig defines health to be a perfect equilibrium of all the functions of the body—where the balance between waste and supply is faithfully kept up; which, to our modern and homely way of thinking and expressing ourselves, is as much as to say, a man is in health when he is well. Disease, of course, is the opposite condition to this, where the equilibrium is disturbed, when there

* Called, in medical language, Eremacausis.

necessarily follows some change of structure, however small. The positive disorganization may not be easily recognizable, if at all—but it *must* occur. Every atom of the body has its office, and its function depends upon its property, and where is there a particle without one?

A ripple in the silent pool from the falling of a pebble extends its circles to its confines, in relation to the force of the agitation, and so it is with the dissemination of disease.

Health may be likened to a summer's day—disease may be compared to a shower or a storm, and the mischief and danger depend upon the violence and permanence of either. Notwithstanding the figurative language, this flourish about a definition—the comparison is a simple one, and when admitted, leads a man to think where the evil lies, and what it is; thus, then, do we arrive at the understanding of the problem just given. Disease, like the pebble thrown in the pool, extends its disturbance far and wide, and hence the shock of an upset stomach to the whole system, or a gouty toe to the generation of fever—by *sympathy*, which is the exercise of a law, as the ripple on the water.

The practice of medicine hitherto certainly has had the odium of being considered more or less entirely empirical; but not a medicine is administered now whose operation and influence are not pre-ascertainable, and where a doubt exists, it is because we do not reflect, rather than we cannot find out.

Liebig seems to attribute all diseases to the disordered condition of the blood; and, consequently, we are to infer that the onus of a distemper lies in the food we take, the air we breathe, or the external worldly or the moral circumstances which influence the condition of that fluid; and he further intimates that the cure, therefore, of disease rests less on the chymical properties of drugs than the dieting, nursing, and general regimen, on which the creation of healing blood depends. The *chymical* treatment of disease is rather of a circumscribed nature, being confined to the supply of those elements which enter into the composition of the blood; thus have we recommended the inhalation of oxygen or vital air, as it is called, the internal exhibition of iron, sulphur, lime, soda, iodine, &c.; all others act on the principles of counter-irritants.

The leading elements of the body have been stated to be oxygen, hydrogen, nitrogen, and carbon; this reiteration is imperative to enforce the importance of the following fact:—of these elements, be it remembered, the nitrogen is *the* important inhabitant of the organized structures. Although the other three enter into the composition of man, they only fulfil the purposes of fuel to the vital fire ; the carbon not consumed is stored up for future occasion in appropriate cells, and is denominated fat. The nitrogen that becomes displaced by the new food in the ordinary rule of change passes off by the kidneys and glandular system, or else supplies the place of carbon when that element is deficient, as in the progress of starvation. Liebig considers the brain and nerves to be composed of a somewhat higher organization than that which enters into the formation of the other structures of the body, and that they are less easily arranged. All the more important glandular secretions are, at the expense of the *nitrogen*, the sole support of animal life, and hence, where those secretions are usually profuse, as in the irregularities alluded to in the opening pages of this book, it needs no ghost to point out the fearful consequences, and how and in what manner such drainages act, to the prejudice of those essential portions of our bodies, the brain and nerves ; hence have we the disordered and impaired intellect of early life ; hence the faulty state of our bodily and mental sensations; hence the debility—for what is strength but the full tone of healthy organization, and how can there be tone, when the organization be imperfect ?—what mars the sound of a cracked bell but its fracture ? what robs the musical chord of its full vibratory intonation but laxity in its tension ? and what is debility but incapacity for the muscle to lift its weight, the stomach to furnish its solvent juice, or the brain to be the harbinger of our will and desires ? The excesses of gourmandism, drinking, smoking, and other exhaustive practices, destroy the vital structure, not only by the consumption of its elements, its nitrogen especially, but by impeding the acquisition of oxygen and loading the system with carbon, which accounts for congested livers, diseased respiration, disordered kidneys, and the whole host of diseases abridging or making life miserable.

Of the importance of the other, besides the four leading elements, the physiologist is fully alive. Iron is detected in the blood—phosphorous in the nervous system—lime in the bones and membranes—potass and soda in the secretions, all of which severally play their part.

Notwithstanding the objections which the common-sense man, the hater of all " outlandish names," he who would " call water water, and fire fire," may have to the new vocabulary of terms, to him so mysterious (for as well might an Englishman object to the French and German being different to his native tongue, as to deny to chymistry a language of its own), still a little reflection will reconcile him to his new world of ideas, and the impression will be the more lasting and effective when he thinks in his own tongue, and construes properly the translation I am attempting to give. That man thrives only on elements analogous to those in his self-composition, merely signifies that he should live on nutritious food. Fortunately, Liebig's theory does not alter the arrangement and view given in this book of what we should *eat, drink,* and *avoid*. Butter, sugar, wine, beer, and spirits, although called *non nitrogenized* food, are still known as they are called, and though fattening, palatable, and universally consumed, are *not nutritious ;* and the last three, seemingly strengthening, because stimulating, still in themselves they are not nourishing. They may be strictly called medicinal condiments. Hence, again, not only is innutritious food, unwholesome, not only are excesses in indulgences, in pleasures as they are called, in the overstraining of our appetites, and consequently various powers of life, prejudicial, but equally so are the penalties we impose upon ourselves for such transgressions, namely, the penalty of physic-taking, and when, like the other evils just enumerated, overdone. By physic-taking I apply it in its usual sense—the habit of resorting on nearly all occasions to strong purgative medicines. The weakness and faintness so rapidly consequent upon diarrhœa, or bowel complaint, is well-known ; the frequent, and to some people who take physic all their lives, the continual drainage kept up (such individuals never experiencing a solid evacuation), must be evident, and more so when it is told that each operation is at the expense of not merely the feastings and gorgings of yesterday, but of the principal elements of life—each muscle, each nerve, each sense, gives up a portion of its individual self. Again, the ostensible purpose of such remedies is to dislodge the excess of carbon, but what is the use of so doing if the resupply be immediately at hand ?—the hurtful nature of such violent excesses, of one day draining the system, and the next day filling it to repletion, must be apparent to all who think of it—and the individual, guilty of such ways, lives but too soon to find it out. By the continuance of purgation, at last more carbon is thrown off than received, and the waste of the body then is kept up, at the expense of the nitrogen. A coat worn in all weathers can not last so long as one well taken care of; and it is preposterous to suppose that the body does not wear out—it is true, it is made to last, with care, the often-quoted term of three score and ten, and more, but, like the coat, if subjected to undue vicissitudes it cannot possibly exist half its time.

The practice of giving purgative medicines in almost every disease, is a leading feature in physic—medical men resort to it—some make it their hobby—the public seem intuitively to imitate them. The poor man flies to his dose of salts, while he who is disinclined for such and similar drinks, swallows some quack pill. Purgatives are the bases of nearly all the quack medicines. Occasional purgation is indispensable; but how much better would it be to withhold the excess poured into the system, and to suffer nature to get rid of its natural quantity in the natural way! Physic (purgative) is, at best, when even properly and skilfully administered, but a necessary evil.

Ill health assumes many very formidable aspects, and the moment a man falls ill, he loses courage, and flies to physic: it is a popular saying, that a stitch in time saves nine; but then finding relief once, he resorts to it again and again, and having discovered, as he fancies, the remedy, he returns to the cause of his disease.

The folly of taking physic indiscriminately (quack medicines, for instance) is so glaring, that no man in his senses would risk the danger. Surely, the proper person to repair a watch is not the dressmaker, and how can any one dare to say that this or that medicine will cure all disorders, any more than the milliner would insist that she was the proper person to mend a broken spring of a chronometer or the wheel of a stage coach? The principles of physic may be learned by the divine, as well as music by the amateur; but principles without practice seldom lead to perfection, and the dabblers in physic, the pill-mongers, and the nostrum-venders, are sad outrages upon the present state of society.

Finally, to recapitulate. The body consists of elements, derivable only from food, analogous to itself in elementary composition.

The main structures of the body—the blood, the brain, and nervous system, and the substantiality of man—are made up of nitrogenized atoms. Other elements are present, such as oxygen, hydrogen, and carbon; but they are principally designed to form the fluids of the body, and to preserve its heat. Their undue proportion constitutes disease. Their equalization rests upon the supply and their combustion; judgment and the will can regulate the former, and fresh air and exercise the latter. The administration of physic is a science; judiciously exercised, the due and proper proportion of the elements of the body can be preserved; obnoxious ones can be removed, and those necessary, furnished.

The treatment of ill-health by diet and regimen, is really very simple, ay, and very beautiful.

There is no doubt but that, owing to diet and regimen, we are indebted for all those qualities that make man the noble fellow he is. The clear head, the strong arm, the bright eye, the fair skin, and the due, universal energy, are we bound to give credit for, to the care a man takes of himself, supposing the notion to be followed out from parent to son; and we may depend upon it, in like manner have we to thank ourselves for feeble and enervated health, for listless and tamed subjection, and for indifference, at last, to our actual existence.

The inferences to be gathered from Liebig's theory are, that we should rather support than debilitate—that we should refrain rather than overfeed; and the main and most effective proposition contained in it, is, that we should study "*How to live,*"—that we should really eat and drink upon principle, as we would fill any other office in life. The stores are so abundant for our delight and downright enjoyment, that the selection to secure health is not confined to those which are insipid or tasteless. Man may even be luxurious—be an epicure, and yet gain health and strength at every meal. The hurtful things in this life are not those which are the nicest, but which the vitiated taste of man and the novelty of enjoyment provoke.

If my reader have journeyed with me thus far, I shall be content if I have even excited in him a curiosity to extend the inquiry concerning himself. The theory of Liebig involves a subject that, when more generally understood, cannot fail to be as generally appreciated. The chymistry of man, if investigated, will be more likely to enable him to "know himself," as the Scripture adviseth, than all the closet meditations which logicians or moral philosophers can advise upon.

There is in this country a disinclination to attach the full importance to organic or physical health, lest the idea savor or seem to encourage the atheistical doctrines of materiality; but the surmise is false. The modifications of light are owing to the medium through which it is transmitted, and the manifestations of the mind are in like manner marked by the organization which exhibits it.

It may well be said, how fearfully and wonderfully we are made; but complicated and mysterious as the whole fabric seems to be, yet how beautiful is the arrangement! The ingenuity of man could not suggest a single improvement! Not a fibre, or vein, or artery, have we superfluous—not an atom is wanting.

CHAPTER VIII.

REMARKS ON BATHING GENERALLY.

On Warm Bathing.

READER, did you ever take a warm bath? The question may be libellous, and yet no more than asking you whether you have ever been to Paris. Formerly, the latter was an adventure, and a remarkable one, in our history; and scarcely less so was the former. There was, however, some justifiable excuse for not bathing; bathing-houses were few, and bathing was expensive; consequently a general tepid wash was rarely indulged in, as we grew beyond the nursery Saturday nights' ablutions. But let us move the original question, and if the answer be in the negative, let me suggest the experiment. *Take one.* Apart from its cleanly properties, its moral virtues, and its salutary tendency, it has a strong inducement in the personal comfort which it affords. Supposing you never took one, to induce you to do so, fancy for a moment the delight of warmth. Standing with your back to the fire is proverbial; warming our hands before the blazing coal is a luxury in cold weather; shaving in hot weather—what a pleasure! Taxing also our memory for our last cold; was not half the cure of it effected by the hot foot-bath, by which the shrivelled skin, the bound head, and the lazy back-ache, were resolved into soft and refreshing sleep? Now fancy the entire body immersed, neck high, in a warm bath. Even the dumb must speak in its praise. First, we will consider it as a luxury; secondly, a remedy; lastly, a duty.

Enjoyments are better appreciated by contrasts. Take, for instance, arriving at the end of a journey, "nipped to the nose," fingers cold as icicles, toes senseless as marble, teeth chattering upon a still tongue, and the body trembling, shivering, and fluttering, like a poor dog rescued from drowning, and withal exhausted by, most likely, wakefulness, possibly wet, and fatigue: imagine or recollect all these phenomena, and then remember the elysium of a hot-bath, if you happen to have entered one; or, if such a fact cannot be recalled, should the like feelings ever assail you again, in justice to my commendation, *try one.* It surpasses the toasting before the kitchen fire; an oven bears no comparison to it, and bed is a sorry rival. Such a state of things as half-freezings, and similar sufferings, are highly dangerous; and a cold caught one day often sees the victim coffined in a week. A hot bath, taken at the fitting moment, arrests the threatened invasion, dissolves the frigid members, reanimates noes, fingers, and toes, sends the blood merrily on to every extremity, where ten minutes before it was a stranger, and composes the body in a state of thankful and grateful ease, and sends death about his business. This is not a mere fanciful sketch by a bath proprietor, but a positive and undeniable truth; and a warm bath aptly taken has, in hundreds of instances, and thousands too, averted and cured illnesses that bitter experience tells have proved fatal for the want of one. A cold is the most accessible of all complaints in this variable climate; neglected, it leads to the most fatal. *A warm bath is the readiest, cheapest, quickest, best, and most certain cure.* I am not the only authority for the assertion. Every travelled man of forty can attest it; "*Probatum est!*" Now, setting aside this rhapsody on the best way of warming ourselves, and of killing a cold, the reader may desire to know what medical men think of the virtues and usefulness of warm bathing. That it is conducive to health; that it absolutely is the best substitute for exercise and physic, when the former can scarcely be had, and of the latter there be too much already swallowed, is indisputable. That it equalizes the circulation of the blood; renders the skin supple and moist; promotes free perspiration, and relieves the body from a layer of thick, obstructive accumulation of scurf, and oleaginous surfacial deposit, and so proves salutary, giving thereby an impetus to absorption and secretion, is also a great fact, and, therefore, it is most wholesome and wise, on not too frequent occasions, to avail of it.

A man calling himself in health, to keep himself so, should certainly take a warm bath once a week throughout his life; certainly a fortnight should not pass without one. Let the skeptic try the experiment, and, in addition to improved feelings, the great one of knowing his entire body to be clean, and spotless, and wholesome, will be such a comfort, that a misery is in store if the practice be omitted. The effect of a warm bath to a person in health, is highly delightful. The sensations during the process are exquisite, and afterward no less so. The liberty of motion, the pleasurable and agreeable diffusion of warmth, and the perfect ease during the indulgence, have no parallel. The flexibility of the joints, the freedom of respiration, the improved tone of nervous feeling in mind and body, intellect being brighter, and every faculty livelier—memory, thought and idea at command, after the bath—are notorious truths known to the patron of the warm ablution. The next view may be the virtues of warm bathing in illness, in severe cases, or to a person (for these observations apply to both sexes, and, of the two, with perhaps greater right to the ladies) in delicate health, in dyspeptic health, in nervous health. First, the bath allays all pain, and removes all, not positively inflammatory—and even in these cases is highly serviceable under proper advice; it quiets all nervous irritability; promotes general perspiration; quickens and yet softens the circulation, overcoming thereby obstructions in deep-seated parts, and allowing an easy and regular flow of the blood throughout its course. Warm bathing also acts beneficially on the kidneys and urinary organs; it helps the bowels, and stomach, and liver, giving new life to each, the action of each being thereby healthily excited; it consequently promotes digestion, and contrary to the popular fear of a warm bath, weakening, it in reality strengthens the system; and furthermore, in opposition likewise to the apprehension that a warm bath is dangerous, as being liable to give cold afterward, it, I unhesitatingly declare, fortifies you against one. Colds are only taken when the bath exhausts, when it is taken too hot, or the bather has been too long in it, or he incautiously submits himself to draughts, or may linger about in the cold and damp air, and so "take a chill" on coming out of one. In all cases of restlessness—the figits—in hypochondriasis, better known as low spirits—general bodily and mental depression—the warm bath is most useful; it tranquilizes the whole system, induces a good night's rest, soothes excitability, stills an irregular and fluctuating pulse, and calms a turbulent mind. As a matter of health and duty, the bath is imperative; as one of ease, and comfort, and enjoyment, and lastly, of cleanliness, incomparable; if omitted from distrust, in the first instance, folly; if from dilatoriness or indolence, or on the score of trouble or expense, unpardonable.

The usual temperament of a warm bath is ninety-eight degrees, but according to the object in view, it can be modified and borne at the pleasure of the bather; if taken for mere refreshment and cleanliness, the above heat will prove very agreeable and suitable for the purpose; if suffering from cold or other indisposition, and perspiration be desirable, one hundred degrees will be found effective, and ten minutes are quite long enough to remain in it; if the stay be much protracted, exhaustion follows, and the effect is hurtful. The French people accustom themselves to pass a full hour in the warm bath, but the practice is relaxing, and indeed enervating. The best time for taking a bath is before a meal, or else some time after one. The morning is most favorable for invalids, because the body is fresh and able to encounter any little extra fatigue; but the bath is equally serviceable at all periods of the day, morning, noon, or evening, and those persons whose engagements are imperative, during what are called business hours, must not plead "the fear of taking cold after sunset" as an excuse for the omission. Indeed, the apprehension of taking cold (which prevails to a popular degree), after a warm bath under any circumstances, is quite erroneous; for, in fact, instead of predisposing a person to a catarrh or a rheumatic attack, or, in plain language, a cold, the bath absolutely helps to stave one or either of the others off. The absolute effect of a hot bath is, that it stimulates, arouses, and keeps up the circulation, thereby diffusing warmth throughout the frame, which renders it invulnerable to the dreaded evil; and if a man do not suffer that excitement to subside, and do not linger about in the cold or damp air, but proceed briskly on his way, he will derive the double benefit of feeling stronger and better, if possible, than before, and of enjoying the refreshment of the immersion. A bath may be taken safely in the "bitterest" and coldest weather. Foggy and damp, and wet days are the least favorable for the indulgence. In the summer the bath is most essential, for the skin having double duty to perform, it urgently requires to be kept cleanly, lest any obstruction to the perspiration should ensue. If the bath be wanted for a specific purpose, and the illness be one of uncertainty, or beyond the comprehension of the invalid, a medical opinion had better be had; but I am not speaking, "*fee*-prospectively," for, invaluable as professional guidance must be admitted to be, on all and every occasion, especially if it be good, of which I have dilated upon elsewhere, I am an advocate that common sense should tell, not only "when to run for the doctor," but when to do without him, and therefore must leave my readers to discriminate for themselves. Great as the pleasure, delight, and salubrity of a warm bathing is, there is a time and season for all things. I have observed that, for cleanliness, and comfort, and health, a warm bath may be taken once a week, or once a fortnight at least, but for special purposes, one may be taken daily for a time, or twice or thrice a week; but the practice must not degenerate into such frequency as to enervate and enfeeble, which, like any other practice carried to excess, it will do. All that I can add is, that the warm bath is a most excellent adjunct in the cure and maintenance of health. It rarely disagrees, but its services are manifold, and the introduction of baths for the poor is a noble national donation, and will doubtless tend to the extension of the practice of ablution ; for cleanliness is a speaking advertisement, and carries with it the comforts, agreeable feelings, and permanent health, which warm bathing can so effectively administer.

On Vapor, Sulphur, Fumigating, and other Bathing.

Vapor bathing is an immense luxury and a vastly powerful remedial agent. Its story is soon told. The bather is closeted in a chamber, like a tent, which is furnished with fragrant steam, which quickly surrounds the body, and soon causes great but bearable warmth that ends in profuse perspiration. The feelings on the occasion are most delightful ; a vapor bath has been fancifully compared to " Mahomet's seventh heaven." It is needless to go into long details here ; but I may briefly enumerate the many complaints, vapor, fumigating, heated air, or other medicated bathing, triumphs over. The various baths of this kind are to suit special local diseases and the constitutions of particular individuals ; but they had all better (the baths) be taken (more or less) under medical surveillance. First and foremost it may be stated that few skin complaints yield without the use of the bath. Some of the more inveterate kinds admit of no other remedy. All chronic painful affections, such as exist in the bones, joints especially, the broad muscles of the back, the thick muscles of the buttocks, thighs, constituting lumbago, rheumatism, neuralgia, &c., all more or less modifications of the same malady, are ameliorated and cured by medical bathing. The vapor bath is an almost infallible cure for a cold. This and the warm bath may honestly be called the hot-water cure. It is greatly useful in chronic affections of the kidneys, in nervous affections of the various parts of the body—tic doloreux especially—and also as a great renovator of health, inducing a healthful action upon the circulation, provoking the proper functions of the liver and digestive organs, the skin, and all the various secretions. Steam bathing constitutes a system in itself, and is worthy of every reliance and attention on the part of the profession and the public ; but theory will help very little either party. I have witnessed the effects of bathing on a very large scale, both in England, and at the " Hôpital St. Louis" in Paris, where I saw many hundreds of cures of skin and other diseases effected by bathing ; and I therefore can confidently affirm that bathing such as I have enumerated, and its many modifications, must be seen to be understood, when it will be found to be a great medical agent, and to supersede a vast deal of the drugging and physicking poor human mortality is driven to have recourse to.

On Cold Bathing.

This work being professedly "A Guide to Health," it would be very imcomplete, having introduced the subject of warm bathing, did I not say a word or two on its friendly antagonist, cold bathing; for, strange to say, although apparently of such a dissimilar nature, its tendency and usefulness are the same. "The Cold-Water cure" has made a great stir in the world; and it is ridiculous to suppose, notwithstanding the prejudices against it among certain medical men and others who know nothing about it, that it is a mere chimera, when thousands of people recover and live to tell of the immense service it has rendered them. No matter whether the cure has been effected by temperate living and by country exercise, certain it is, invalids who have employed cold bathing in conjunction, as far as they can judge by their own feelings, and as far as observers can declare from personal knowledge—certain it is that cold bathing, either local or general, is a highly important remedy, and that by its means the parties in question have got well. Physic, without the observance of careful living, exercise, and fresh air, and other such adjuncts, would do very little alone; but the credit is usually given to the medicine, and why should not the bath be as fairly treated? *The cold shower bath, the douche bath,* where a large stream of cold water is forcibly directed to particular parts of the body, have severally their patrons. *The sitz bath,* similar to the common hip bath, but not so deep, is really a great agent in diseases of the pelvic viscera, or organs contained in the lower part of the abdomen, and in nervous affections, pains, and debility of the neighboring structures, female complaints, &c. *The cold plunge bath,* although taken, perhaps, more for pastime than health, yields both. Mark the color and glow of the bather after a jump-in, a short swim, and a quick dressing;—consult his feelings the remainder of the day and he will tell you the bath strengthens him, cheers his spirits, gives him a freshness of feeling unattainable by any other means; that, in fact, he longs for the next morning to give him his next immersion. Why do people congregate by the seaside and there venture among the sportive waves, allowing the foaming sea to engulph them, were they not convinced they derived benefit from the practice? Young and old, after a sojourn, even though it be brief, at the coast, return home renovated and replenished with healthful and happy looks, and the majority will speak with rapture of the benefits of sea-bathing. Indeed, the fact is incontrovertible. Of course, cold bathing, in all its forms, requires some little prudence in its indulgence. It is not wise to remain in too long, nor can it be done with impunity any more than in the warm bath (two errors of frequent happening), and therefore certain rules should be observed as a guidance; for instance, except an immediate reaction follows the immersion, the shock of the bath leaves behind a chill which may end in a severe cold, or establish rheumatism, or set up fever or general irritability and it may thereby weaken instead of strengthening the bather It is therefore prudent to jump in, move about for a couple of minutes, come out and dress, and then walk about to keep up the excitement. The best time for bathing is the morning, either before or after breakfast—before, if strong enough, or an hour after breakfast; if the former time prove not so salutary, cold bathing tells its effects very speedily; if it disagree, the sensations will bespeak as much; if on the contrary, the desire to repeat it will predominate. The bath should never be taken on a full stomach: and it is unwise to compel young people to bathe against their inclinations. Diffidence may be overcome, but dread, if defied, may produce illness. Bathers must in all instances, be guided by their feelings when and how often they may take the baths; but they may safely venture every or every other morning. The cold shower bath may be taken every morning all the year round, and some people take the same evenings also, and with benefit. The sitz and douche had better be taken under medical guidance. The temperature (for that varies, owing to weather, situation, &c.,) must be studied. Some weak systems can not command a wholesome and prompt reaction from a *very* cold bath, and therefore the bath should be changed for a tepid; but the ordinary cold bath in the summer season, as at the sea, is about the most agreeable and safe. In conclusion, cold water, whether in tub, stream, or sea, is one of those beneficent gifts Nature has bestowed on man for his own use, and, if employed with careful consideration, affords the end in view—universal good,—and can not but elicit from every thankful mind the homage and gratitude due to the great and benevolent Author of its source.

www.ingramcontent.com/pod-product-compliance
Lightning Source LLC
Chambersburg PA
CBHW020144170426
43199CB00010B/878